Touch and Emotion in Manual Therapy

For Rachel

For Churchill Livingstone:

Editorial Director, Health Sciences: Mary Law
Project Manager: Ewan Halley
Project Development Editor: Valerie Dearing
Design Direction: Judith Wright

Touch and Emotion in Manual Therapy

Bevis Nathan DO MA
Registered Osteopath

Foreword by

Leon Chaitow DO ND
Practitioner and Senior Lecturer, Centre for Community Care and
Primary Health,
University of Westminster, London, UK

Photographs by

Sandra Lousada

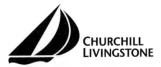
CHURCHILL
LIVINGSTONE

EDINBURGH LONDON NEW YORK PHILADELPHIA SAN FRANCISCO
SYDNEY TORONTO 1999

CHURCHILL LIVINGSTONE
An imprint of Harcourt Brace and Company Limited

© Harcourt Brace and Company Limited 1999
© Photographs: Sandra Lousada 1999

⚓ is a registered trademark of Harcourt Brace and Company Limited

First published 1999

ISBN 0443 056579

British Library of Cataloguing in Publication Data
A catalogue record for this book is available from the British Library.

Library of Congress Cataloging in Publication Data
A catalog record for this book is available from the Library of Congress.

Medical knowledge is constantly changing. As new information becomes
available, changes in treatment, procedures, equipment and the use of
drugs become necessary. The editors/authors/contributors and the
publishers have, as far as it is possible, taken care to ensure that the
information given in this text is accurate and up to date. However,
readers are strongly advised to confirm that the information, especially
with regard to drug usage, complies with latest legislation and standards
of practice.

The
publisher's
policy is to use
**paper manufactured
from sustainable forests**

Printed in China
NPCC/01

Contents

Foreword

Honouring the mind, and the intimate connections it has with the state of the body, is a concept which attracts a great deal of lip-service from practitioners and therapists of all schools. It has become the defining central feature of the concept of holism, of consideration of the 'whole person'. But just how widely is this apparent embracing of an idea put into practice, and how well are its full implications really understood by those who use manual methods to address the pain and distress of their patients?

When we touch someone we do more than apply a physical, mechanical contact. Certainly, we often use touch in a technical, investigative, actively 'doing' manner but, when we do, whether we are aware of it or not, what we are doing also has a psychologically significant content. Any manual therapist or practitioner who operates (or who attempts to operate) on a purely biomechanical level may achieve good results in instances where a problem is almost exclusively (if anything ever is) the result of mechanical strain or trauma. However, when the body-mind link is neglected the multi-dimensional possibilities which exist become uni-dimensional. So, it is reasonable to ask, would it not be better to understand and apply bodywork's potentials in a more rounded way? This book provides the intellectual and practical framework of understanding from which such an exercise can emerge.

In essence, what Nathan unveils is the often neglected aspect of manual medicine in which psychologically significant touching of a therapeutic nature is inherent in what therapists do, whether they acknowledge this or not.

Bevis Nathan argues for a comprehensive approach to the patient and challenges bodyworkers to expand their horizons by reviewing what it is they are actually doing. By taking a broader look at what at first may appear to be purely biomechanical mechanisms a more powerful potential should emerge.

There are many practitioners and therapists who seem to shield themselves intellectually from 'heart-based' definitions of what they are doing by using mechanical, procedural, structural models (and language) to explain their work. This text strongly suggests that such approaches fail to truly deal with the whole person and that treating people instead of bodies, or parts of bodies, requires a far greater understanding of the individual than is common or current in most branches of manual medicine. While expressive, thoughtful touch incorporates technical, mechanical, procedural methods, all such methods contain psychological implications, which Nathan reveals and cogently discusses.

In this important book, the author takes us on a practical and philosophical exploration which reinforces the importance of recognising both the physiological and psychological impact of touch on homeostatic mechanisms. Part of the association between the mind and the physical body is shown to relate to the role of muscles as sensory organs, making the sensations they produce emotionally significant or, as the author puts it, 'the emotions themselves' – with powerful physical sensations often accompanying particular emotions – pleasant and unpleasant.

Quite logically, Nathan then looks through the other end of the telescope, suggesting that, if bodywork can be seen to influence emotional states, psychotherapy should be able to influence effectively many of the problems which manual therapists are asked to treat. Indeed, he contends that muscular hypertonia is largely caused by centrally ordered psychological processes – except in the case of obvious tissue damage. The need for all manual medicine therapists and practitioners to have a greater understanding of psychology is implicit in this broad model, as is the need for psychotherapists to have a greater understanding of the physical body and manual medicine.

In the end, this intellectually challenging yet satisfying and highly practical book is a plea for a wider interpretation, and greater understanding, of what manual practitioners and therapists can do, and for as great a degree of integration of mind and bodywork as possible. As someone who started out on the professional journey with a largely mechanistic viewpoint but who has been moulded by experience to recognise the absolute necessity for an emotional, psychological (often central) dimension in bodywork, the author offers this book as a powerful validation and provides many new areas to explore.

Leon Chaitow

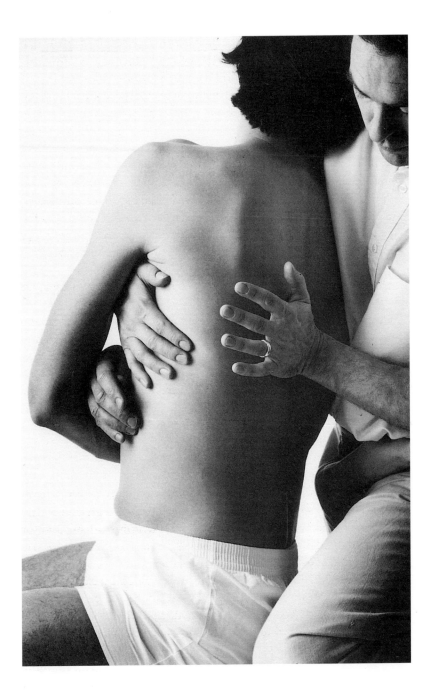

Preface

This book is written for manual practitioners in the orthodox field of medicine, primarily for those practitioners who manipulate the body — that is chiropractors, osteopaths and physiotherapists. It should also be of interest to all health care professionals who touch people in the context of caring or healing (doctors, nurses, masseurs, aromatherapists, practitioners of therapeutic touch, etc.).

What actually happens when manual practitioners touch their patients? If we ask people the question, 'are they manipulating bodies or persons?', most of them will answer 'bodies', because this seems obvious. To say that practitioners are manipulating persons perhaps implies they are in some way altering patients' psychological processes, and that might seem unreasonable, even unethical.

On the other hand, can we really separate people from their bodies? Ask yourself, are you separate from your body? Is it you who is running or is it your body? Did you cut yourself yesterday or was that your body you cut? There is an area of ambiguity. Yes, you cut yourself, and it was your arm that you cut. Yes, you are running, and we can safely say that your legs are doing most of the work. What this superficial analysis reveals is that generally we say it is ourselves, as persons, who are experiencing these things, but when we want to be anatomically specific, for whatever reason, we talk about parts of our bodies. When we do this the parts seem to become our possessions — merely objects — and no longer our*selves*. Conceptually, we are able to separate ourselves from our bodies.

Similarly, if we manipulate a patient's lumbar spine, or massage his shoulders, he can experience *himself* as being massaged or manipulated, and also his *shoulders* or *back* as being massaged or manipulated.

Returning to the original question of whether practitioners are manipulating bodies or persons — what are the implications of each answer?

■ I am manipulating this body. Technically, I need to be very skilful, and I need to be sensitive to the qualities of the underlying tissue, using just the right amount of force. I don't need to speak, but I need to be acutely aware of the potential for causing discomfort. I test the movement characteristics after the treatment is over. There, that seems better. Now I'll hand the body back to the person and say 'How do you feel?'

■ I am manipulating Mrs Jones. I keep in mind what I might be experiencing if I were her. The same technical skill is necessary, the same tissue sensitivity. I realise that Mrs Jones will feel differently about my touching different areas of her body, and she will feel differently about my touching the same areas of her body in different ways. She might not like that technique, but when I do this one she says, 'Oh that feels like just what I need'. I realise that Mrs Jones wouldn't let me do this if I were not qualified and in a health care setting because she has very few clothes on and is being totally passive. She allows me to manipulate her as I see fit after I have briefly explained what I am about to do and why. I know that she thinks her body is unsightly because she has told me so. I therefore feel that my manipulation, by touching most parts of her body (limbs, head, neck, back, sternum, rib-cage, abdomen, pelvic bones), imparts to her a sense of being valued and accepted, even if this is only recognised unconsciously. I also expect some patients — and Mrs Jones might be one of them — to have an improved body image after treatment. Such patients believe that before treatment they were in some sense not quite right, and that after treatment this has been corrected. Furthermore, I remember that when I was a student I stretched a patient's lumbar spine by curling him up into a fetal ball and holding him there with a slight rocking motion for half a minute. A favourite tutor and colleague said to me, 'The last person who did that to him was his mother'. I therefore bear in mind that some techniques invoke body-memory of primal, physical experiences of loving, conveyed by 'containing' touches. They may also evoke memories of physical abuse.

It is clear that, of the two scenarios, the second is more ethical, realistic, empathic, human. It is therefore a wiser approach. In this scenario, Mrs Jones's body remains, in the mind of the practitioner, intimately connected with her person throughout the treatment. It is not somehow separated from her during the treatment and then handed back to her after it. In fact the practitioner does not have a

We consider subjects reporting (SOAP) as body symptoms rather than life situation. This is why I said that SOAP are like marginal notes - lifeless abstractions that miss the true subjective.

body in mind but an *embodied person*. By maintaining the attitude that he is treating a particular person, Mrs Jones, rather than just a body, the practitioner remains aware of a further set of parameters which enable the treatment to be more effective. This attitude increases the practitioner's understanding of Mrs Jones's bodily processes because they are placed in the context of Mrs Jones's life. It provides insight into how Mrs Jones expresses herself through her body and also into how she might be suffering.

However, despite the fact that a manual practitioner might keep Mrs Jones's self in view, rather than just her body, Mrs Jones is free to decide for herself when it is her body that is being treated and when it is her self ('that *bit*'s so sore', or 'you're hurting *me*'; and '*it* moves more easily now', or '*I* feel freer'). This is because she has been taught, by medicine, science and our society, to separate her body from herself in a variety of situations. One of the advantages of this is that, for example, when she visits a physician for an internal examination it is less embarrassing because the physician is performing a procedure on a part of her body, rather than doing something incredibly intimate and invasive to *her*. It is true of course that the intimacy and invasiveness still exist, but awareness of this is suppressed in order to render the situation more bearable. *[missing her internal experience]* *[separating the body from the self]*

But what are the implications of this separation for manual medicine? Rather than saying 'I have felt so uptight and constricted in my life recently', I might say 'my neck and back have been so terribly tight recently'. Perhaps if I recognise bodily tightness and constriction as being attributes of myself, then, with a little reflection, I would gain insight into those aspects of my life that are uncomfortable. I would learn how I am reacting to life physically and emotionally. It is, after all, the unconscious aspects of the central nervous system that are responsible for postural muscular hypertonia. If, on the other hand, I keep tightness and constriction firmly located in my body — the machine — then a mechanic is what is called for. I may never realise the extent to which my body reliably reflects my attempts to integrate my environment, my relationships, my thoughts and feelings. *[body as truth teller]* *[unconscious]*

Most manual practitioners who touch patients do so with the general assumption that a human body can be likened to a sophisticated machine, and most patients also hold the same view. This view *[Medicine]*

We meet the Designer thru his work i the body

I hope he is not a Reichian!

xiv PREFACE

causes two problems. First, it overlooks any explicit psychological significance in dealing directly and intimately with patients when using manipulative therapy (although it is by no means invariably useful or appropriate to consider these). Second, it prevents patients from realising and acting upon the extent of the somatic effects of their lives' experiences. These effects are not normally considered the province of human life in general because they are traditionally allocated to merely mechanical realms — the body/machine irritatingly fails us from time to time. In fact it is probable that the body-as-machine view causes repression of important emotional and even existential issues which are acutely relevant to the life and health of patients. Such repressed issues may surface during manual practitioners' intimate contact with patients.

The 'intimacy' which, according to this book, exists between interpersonal touch and personal emotional issues means that it is high time the body-as-machine view was put aside while the full scope and pertinence of these psychological realities are thoroughly researched. In many cases the purely physiological rationales which are currently used to explain how manual therapy works are likely to be of questionable importance relative to certain psychological effects. For example, prolonged rhythmic and deep touching, rubbing and holding — so common in manual medicine — will resonate with early body-memories of emotional and physical maternal nurturing. Such techniques will tend to enhance a patient's self-image, and generate pleasure and a sense of being valued and directly healed.

Much attention is currently being paid to the concept of how to deal with patients as people rather than as diseases or bodies. Thus far this preface may seem like an introduction to yet another book dealing with whole-person medicine as it might be applied to manual therapy. But it is different in one very important respect; the subject matter is touch itself — the human significance of touch in the deepest possible sense. Looking at the vast majority of literature in the field of manual therapy, much of it excellent, there is a significant gap; an indispensable sub-subject is conspicuous by its absence. If the constitution of a human being is essentially mind and body, then the missing subject would be psychology — the 'science of the psyche'. The science of the body is already dealt with in glorious detail. The fact that these

The science of the psyche

may be artificial separations does not excuse the popular tendency to ignore one half. In order to show that it is necessary (and not merely interesting) for manual practitioners to study psychological subjects, it must be possible to demonstrate that such necessity follows from a consideration of what manual practitioners actually do. *- Table Talk*

This book therefore deals with the relationship between touching and emotions and is largely devoted to pointing out that when we touch people — whether or not we intend to heal them — it is always psychologically significant. The book contains the evidence and arguments for this premise and begins to explore the consequences for practitioners. One of the most useful outcomes of a consideration of this subject is that it enlarges the practitioner's ethical awareness — a necessary condition for effective, satisfying work.

The word 'emotion' has been used here as a blanket term to include a wide spectrum of affective phenomena, including feelings, attitudes, sentiments and so on. These are commonly said to be 'felt', as opposed to those largely unfelt psychological events such as thoughts, intellectual arguments, decisions and conclusions. I recognise that such separations and definitions beg further questions, but hold that they are acceptable for the purposes of this book's argument.

Bath 1998   Bevis Nathan

Acknowledgements

I am grateful to all patients, colleagues and teachers, past and present, but especially Jacqueline Dunell, Martyn Evans, Kathryn Keuls, Philip Latey, Eyal Lederman, John Meffan, Martin Pascoe, Peter Randell and Stephen Tyreman. Special thanks and love to Liz Fost, James Hawkins, Robin Herbert and Sandra Lousada. Huge thanks to Alex and Val Hackel. Thank you Rachel, Gabriel and Charis for giving me the space.

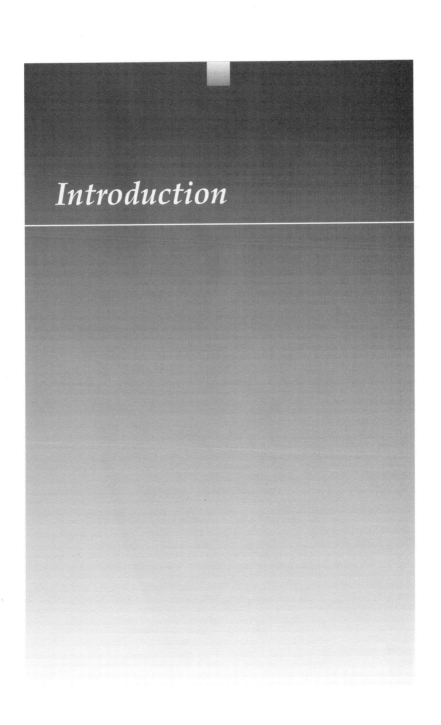

Introduction

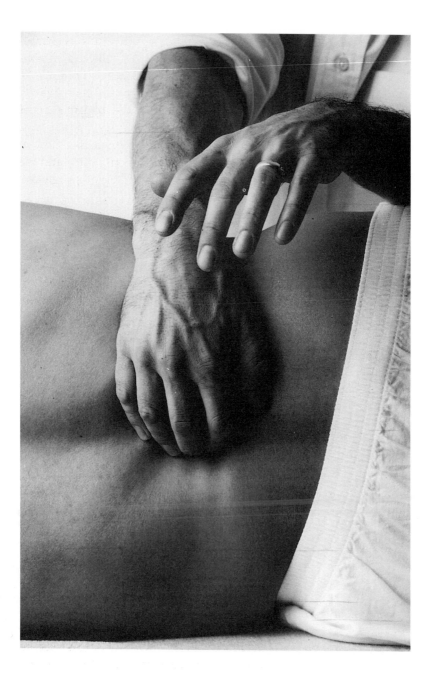

The mood of health care is moving with much momentum away from high-technology, pharmacological, invasive, paternalistic and non-intimate medicine towards a more patient-centred, whole-person approach. This approach recognises the importance of the patient's participation in decision-making, and that of the patient's belief system and attitude in influencing the 'natural history' of an illness. The huge success of the major complementary medicines has, in addition to pointing to some dissatisfaction with orthodoxy and the restraints placed upon its delivery, demonstrated patients' recognition of the value of human interaction in healing.

Touching with intent to heal has an ancient pedigree. Originally an instinctive act based upon compassion and a sense of fraternity, the manipulative therapies have tried to turn it into a scientifically respectable discipline — with a certain degree of success. But in doing so, some of them are in danger not only of failing to form a complete, integral picture of their art, but also of misunderstanding many patients and their real needs.

Osteopathy, chiropractic and physiotherapy are systems of manual diagnosis[1] and treatment of bodily disorders; they lay emphasis on the structural or biomechanical features of such disorders. They rely upon the assumption that the body has mechanical attributes, so that many mechanically defined disorders can be rectified by manual therapy. In this respect they do not differ from orthopaedic surgery and other therapeutic modalities which stress the structural and mechanical components of disease processes.

One of the main features of British[2] osteopathy and chiropractic which set them apart from physiotherapy[3] is that, together with certain views of the body's organisational characteristics, the treatment is exclusively manual (there are a few exceptions to this rule). But in each of these disciplines, and to an even greater extent in therapeutic massage, treatment sessions are long (averaging 30 minutes) and often involve the practitioner's touching much of the patient's exposed body.

Touching a person's body in a non-therapeutic context is not normally considered an act of mainly mechanical significance. Nor is it a proce-dure or a technique — rather it is an act of self-expression, or occasionally self-assertion or preservation. In the main, frequent touching is reserved for parent–child relationships, lovers and close friends. In these contexts it both signifies emotional intimacy and is emotionally significant. Hence, most touching that patients will have experienced is non-healing in intent and is emotionally charged, often at an unconscious level.

This everyday kind of touching is concerned with relationships between people — whole persons — whereas influencing the rationales both for orthodox medicine and for manual therapy in general is mind/body dualism. Because the body is considered more easily investigated than the mind, and its disorders so much more obvious, the assumption is that it is the body which, by and large, manifests disorder and disease. The person appears not to be considered significantly involved. This assumption, currently something of a cliché, has led medicine to focus its chemical and physical therapeutic aims on the body rather than on the person. It has resulted in many astounding successes and many spectacular failures.

The resurgence of interest in holistic approaches to health care is an attempt to heal this apparent breach in orthodox medical thinking, and holistic principles are now being taught in schools of manipulative medicine with fervour. (In fact, it is likely that many medical and paramedical educational institutions have stressed the holistic approach to patient care for decades without having actually deployed the term 'holistic'.) However, relatively little attention has been paid by these professions to the full significance of touching. The manipulative rationale omits from both patient-centred and mechanistic descriptions, that most personal and intimate form of communication, the touch itself. This is probably because in attempting to provide 'acceptable' mechanistic explanations of manipulative healing, it has become blinded to the obvious. In taking for granted the very fact of its manual emphasis, manual therapy is missing the wood whilst down among the physiological trees. The 'wood' is that manual therapy is probably *the* whole-person therapeutic modality *par excellence*.

This book attempts to expose the emotional and psychological issues around touching, and suggests that they are acutely relevant to any manual therapy encounter. They are especially relevant where there is much touching, holding, and rhythmic work, and where the touches show great variation in depth. The book concludes that the use of manual touch as a healing mode should be explored for its psychotherapeutic,[4] in addition to its mechanistic significance.

NOTES

[1] Physiotherapy has progressed from being a medical adjunct to more a complete system. In the past, physiotherapists were expected to comply with a physician's diagnosis and therapeutic recommendation, whereas it is currently common practice for members of this profession to diagnose and treat patients as they see fit (see Chapter 2 of Refshauge & Gass 1995).

[2] The political and clinical situation with respect to osteopathy in North America is quite different from that in the UK. Manipulation is indispensable to British osteopathy and is largely carried out by practitioners not trained in the mainstream medical system. In North America, osteopathy has been absorbed into orthodox medicine and thus surgical and pharmacological intervention are considered within a framework of osteopathic philosophy. Such intervention is thus deemed 'osteopathic'.

[3] This distinction is made because currently only a minority of physiotherapists are trained in manipulation. Together with the increasing use of technology in physiotherapy interventions, this has meant that the emphasis on manual therapy is currently not stressed in this profession as it used to be, and as it is in chiropractic and osteopathy. *PSYCHOTHERAPEUTIC*

[4] This word is being used in at least two senses; firstly to indicate that the efficacy of manual therapy might be partially explained by the positive effect that appropriate treatment has upon those psychological events determining pathophysiological (and healthy) somatic characteristics. Secondly, it is to suggest that manual therapy can be, in a general sense, therapeutic to the psyche (which in this definition includes the body of emotions and volitions in addition to intellectual/cognitive functions).

REFERENCE

Refshauge K M, Gass E M (eds) 1995 Musculoskeletal physiotherapy. Butterworth Heinemann, Oxford

1

Exposing the questions

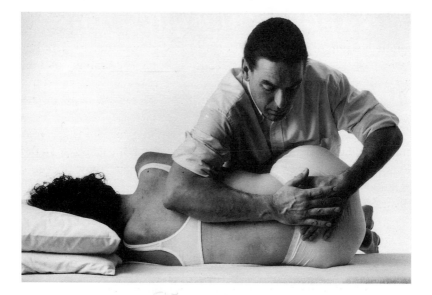

WHAT HAPPENS WHEN YOU TOUCH SOMEONE?

Two sorts of touch experience

Let us suppose a practitioner is performing a gentle technique on a patient's head — a technique intended to cause a therapeutic physiological change to occur in a tissue system in the head. Suppose this procedure is called a 'lateral fluctuation' technique. It involves very gentle holding of the parietal areas of the skull while the patient lies face up on the couch, and is intended to encourage involuntary motion according to a certain pattern. Later in the session, the practitioner decides to perform a longitudinal soft-tissue stretch technique on the patient's low back muscles while the patient lies face down.

The practitioner is performing manipulative procedures, concentrating on her technique and carefully monitoring the response in the living tissues beneath her hands. But the patient's perception of events is quite different. During the first technique she experiences herself as being held and cradled, directly healed. During the second technique, she experiences herself as being caressed, stroked and soothed.

Why are these two experiences of touching so different? From the point of view of the practitioner, the touch is essentially a technique and is analogous to a delicate and skilful engineering procedure. The intention of this touch is to create a therapeutic physiological event in the tissues of the patient, and the rationale underlying the technique is physiological, kinetic or mechanical in nature.

From the patient's point of view, the touch has its roots in non-verbal communication or communion. She does not experience the touch as merely a technique or procedure on her body tissues, it involves her *self*. She is being held, cradled, stroked, caressed, valued, cared-for, *healed*. This patient's experience is above all a psychological and existential one. Indeed, the nature of the events caused by the treatment may well be primarily psychological.

Each patient's experience of touch in manual therapy is individual to them. It will vary from one patient to another and will usually include both types of touch experience. A patient will often have a sense of both the technical manipulation of her body, and also of the caring touch — a physical–empathic communication with herself. The validity and peculiarity of each experience arises as a result of a patient's character, life experiences, and relationship with the practitioner, no less than from the practitioner's technique. Practitioners should remember that in most other areas of a patient's life, cradling or stroking is an act of caring and affiliation, intended to give pleasure or heal.

Two sorts of touch

It is possible to divide touch into two broad categories:

1. touch as a technique or procedure, eg a muscle-stretching manipulation
2. touch as expression, communication, eg hand-holding for comfort.

These two categories of touch usually overlap, so that the specific physiological events in the patient's tissues which the practitioner intends may well be occurring, but at the same time as a unique and unconscious (usually) psychological response. These two types of response are profoundly different in nature. One is mechanical and physiological, the other largely emotional. If most therapeutic touches will evoke emotional responses in addition to mechanical ones, the question arises: which component is responsible for the healing?

What is the relative therapeutic importance of the patient's general sensory–psychological experience compared with the specific physiological effects of the manipulative practitioner's mechanical procedure, and in what way are these two responses related?

Psychological causality

As medical theory matures and as psychology and complementary medicine contribute to this body of knowledge, it is becoming increasingly clear that the psychological inner life of a person is at least as powerful an aetiological factor in disease processes as outer physical and environmental factors. Similarly, this inner life is at least as powerful in healing as forces applied from 'without'. The following abstract, although fictional, is based upon fact.

'*The human body, the human brain, is hard-wired for mystery. You have seen a suffering patient experience profound relief from pain and sleep soundly for the first time in weeks after getting an injection of sterile water, under the impression that it was a potent narcotic. You have seen a patient unable to sit still at the start of an interview leave the examining room calm and placid, simply because the physician has mouthed some meaningless mumbo-jumbo of a diagnosis that sounds impressive and scholarly. You have seen a patient sent for a series of diagnostic X Rays who does not know their purpose but tells the physician later how grateful he is for the relief he has got as a result of the "treatments". And these people do not simply feel better; their pulse goes down, their blood pressure goes down, their serum catecholamines go down, their secretory antibodies go up — their entire body tells us of the power of mystery to heal, and of the terrible harm we will do to those who trust us if we ever try to make too much sense to them.'*
(Brody 1992)

The relative contributions to both pathogenesis and healing from within and from without remain unknown in all but the most obvious cases. In current medical theory, the possibility that disease pathogenesis can result largely from psychological events tends to be put aside. Nevertheless, not only does this possibility remain open, but it is gaining in credibility. Philosophers are divided on whether or not mental causation should be taken seriously, but most regard the arguments against it as weak.

This is not to suggest that the explanations usually offered for the effectiveness of manual medicine are wrong. On the contrary, they are accurate, useful and necessary, but incomplete in so far as they only reveal aspects of the physiological realm. Such explanations concern themselves with only a part of a larger whole which remains incompletely represented in medical literature as a result of a philosophical blind spot.

Meaning — medicine's omission

In common with virtually all medical science, manual therapy is explained in terms that are physiological or mechano-physiological in nature. The final result of a manual technique or a prescribed exercise is interpreted by the discipline of biochemistry. (In cases where this is not strictly true for example when a patient's self-esteem is to be improved by encouraging him to demonstrate for himself his physical ability, it is implicit that this assists or is vital to the healing process). This state of affairs has quite naturally arisen out of the inclusion of manual therapy under the umbrella of medicine, which is mechanistic in nature.

Therapeutic touching in manual medicine is usually described using the same language as descriptions of surgical techniques or pharmacologically induced reactions — as techniques or procedures with mechanical or biochemical effects. But there is something that sets manual therapy apart from many other medical procedures — psychologically meaningful touch. The kind of language common to scientific explanations is inadequate because it is unable to include descriptions of the meaning of touch to patients. The inadequacy of this language may go some way to explain why the notion of a patient's sensory–psychological experience of touch in manual therapy has never been explored for its therapeutic significance (except when labelled as merely placebo).

It is of course true that the experience of therapeutic touching by manual practitioners has never been thought of as contributing seriously to the healing process, largely because of the Cartesian legacy of the body-as-machine view. Such a view does not allow the possibility that mere belief is capable of influencing the course of a disease (even though this view was not Descartes' personal belief).

Why is it vital for theoretical manual therapy to explore touching afresh as a separate subject? Because in so doing it will be possible to avoid the bias intrinsic to a language suitable only for describing the fairly narrow discipline of quantifiable, scientific medicine. Looking at touch as a subject in its own right, theoretical manual medicine will allow it to remain within its larger and proper context, rather than being viewable only through modern medicine's heavily tinted spectacles. It will be more likely to keep in mind the wholeness of the subject — specifically the significance of the experience of being touched in the healing process. The study of touch itself may shed considerable light upon wider issues in the therapeutic process.

CLINICAL EXAMPLES (NON-FICTIONAL)

A. Mechanical technique/head-holding

A patient looked up at her practitioner with tears in her eyes and said 'the head loves being cradled'. The practitioner was performing the lateral fluctuation technique mentioned previously and had been concentrating carefully on her technique. She was unaware of the patient's experience. What a significant statement this was. 'The head' — not 'my head'. To say instead; 'I love it when you cradle my head' would imply an intimate relationship, for cradling the head is an act that has significance outside of manipulative medicine. It can be an act of affection, of healing in the widest sense, or of love. 'I love it when you cradle my head' is clearly an accurate interpretation of the patient's actual words — this is what she really meant. But since it is people and not heads who love, then why did the patient express herself in this particular way?

There are two reasons:

■ First, in order to establish psychological safety. Many patients have good reasons for disguising their feelings, thereby protecting themselves — minimising their vulnerability. In an act of instinctive, habitual self-preservation, the patient projected her love of having her head held and cradled onto her head itself. The head was doing the loving of the cradling — not her. This created a safe boundary between her and the practitioner. She did not admit to the intimacy of the act, which would imply a special relationship between the two *persons* in contact. Instead, she stated the relationship as being between the practitioner and her head — a part of her, a possession, a mere anatomical area which needed 'fixing'. Having avoided any acknowledgement of intimacy, she nevertheless effectively expressed how much she appreciated this particular form of treatment.

■ Second, because most of us behave as if, and believe that our bodies are quite separate from our selves. This belief not only creates the possibility of this patient's projection, but actually encourages it. The separation of bodies from persons is implicit in the Western world view, which has its origin in Platonic times. Western man is increasingly estranged from his body, in parallel with his ever-decreasing direct involvement with nature and his natural, sensual self.

For this patient to admit to the intimacy of the therapeutic encounter might have been psychologically unsafe. Although interpersonal intimacy is not expected in a modern health care setting, it is important to notice that, at least as far as the patient was concerned, intimacy was implicit in the practitioner's act. In the usual form of non-medical transactions, a sensitive, caring, cradling or stroking act would be in the context of compassion. The patient was unaware of any detailed mechanistic explanation of the technique whereby holding someone's head in this specific way produces a therapeutic physiological response. To the patient the treatment did not feel like a medical intervention in the way in which most medical interventions are experienced. It felt instead non-medical, in the same way as a nurse holding a patient's hand during a painful medical procedure is non-medical.

What did this patient need?

The physiological effectiveness of the lateral fluctuation technique can be taken as given. But what must be considered is the probability that this patient needs to be held in order to be healed. It is not enough merely to assume that the mechanical/physiological effects of the lateral fluctuation technique alone are responsible for the totality of the therapeutic effect. Nor is it likely that it is merely these effects which are causing the patient's emotional experience of being cared for. The possibility must be acknowledged that the practitioner need only have placed her hands on the patient's head with due care, refinement of touch, respect and intention to help for such a healing response to be forthcoming.

This kind of healing is reminiscent of the laying on of hands, and the term 'technique' seems somehow inappropriate in this context. It may be the kind of healing that parents give to their small children — rubbing it better, rocking and holding. It is healing, that much is clear, but it is *whole-person* healing and not simply a medical technique or procedure. The medical procedure may also be efficacious, but touching to heal with a physiological rationale is a very modern, Western idea. Human beings have been healing by touching each other in times of physical or emotional distress since time began.

B. Lumbar articulation technique/rocking

A respectable woman in her sixties was being treated for low back pain by a manipulative practitioner. The practitioner had the partially clad woman lie on her side on the treatment couch, with her knees bent up. She placed her thighs against the patient's shins, supported her lumbar spine with both hands, and, leaning over her, squeezed her knees firmly into her abdomen and chest, slowly and rhythmically. After a few repetitions the patient cried 'Oh this is *so* agreeable'. The practitioner was performing a simple lumbar flexion articulation technique. She had been concentrating on achieving an adequate degree of stretch in the posterior lumbar tissues and hip joints, and a rhythm appropriate to the tissue quality. The patient was experiencing *pleasure*. In this instance it is clear that the pleasure was derived at least in part from the contained fetal position, as well as from the rhythmic, rocking motion and the deep stretching of underused postural muscle. She was curled up, held firmly and rocked by her practitioner. The last person to do anything like this to her was probably her mother.

What did this patient need?

If asked to describe the reasons for the improvement in this patient's symptoms, is it justifiable to ignore the positive effects of pleasure? Is it so certain that a physiological rationale for deep muscular stretching and facet joint mobilisation (described as neurovascular events, for example) is an adequate account of what is occurring in this instance?

What are the effects of the technique on the basal ganglia, cerebellum, limbic system and elsewhere? What are the effects on the patient's self-esteem, on her view of her body as being old and without value? What are the effects of stimulating deeply held, preverbal memories of being rocked and cradled by her mother? Or by her late husband? What are the effects of one person merging with another in rhythmic motion, with an attitude of respect, compassion, and intent to heal?

The question again arises, what is it primarily that heals— the technique and its tissue-specific physiological effects or the experience of being held/healed? What is the relationship between the two? Are there any other explanations to which we ought to look for the fullest possible understanding of this interaction?

These questions must be addressed if the theoretical basis of the manipulative therapies is to advance. Without doing so, despite many clinicians' implicit acceptance of relevant psychological realities, it will remain dependent upon incomplete and partitive dogma whilst the body of knowledge of psychosomatic medicine remains largely unused.

EXAMINING THE QUESTIONS MORE CLOSELY

As a reminder, the key questions which this book begins to explore are: What is the relative therapeutic importance of the patient's sensory–psychological experience compared with the specific physiological effects of the manipulative practitioner's mechanical procedures, and in what way are these two things related?

It is assumed in the framing of this question that both the physiological and the psychological effects of touch are capable of causing healing, and that there is a relationship between these two effects.

It is necessary to review briefly why this question arises in the first place. There are many texts that describe or purport to describe the various failures and inadequacies of modern, technological medicine together with their causes, and some of them also describe the great strengths. From out of a general critique, therefore, can be extracted those criticisms that are of particular significance to any argument concerning the psychological significance of therapeutic touching. Two areas of concern are: the limitations of purely physiological descriptions, and the omission of the patient's experience.

Physiological explanations concerning touch

Physiology (*physis* nature + *logos* discourse) is the study of the processes and activities in living beings, especially the study of the functions of the organs and parts during life. This distinguishes it from anatomy (*anatome* dissection) which is the art of dissecting, or artificially separating, the different parts to ascertain position, relations, structure and function. Physiology begins as a branch of biology (for example, when describing the exchanges occurring across a renal reabsorption system). But when it comes down to the level of biochemical processes (for example, when offering an explanation for the activity of sodium ions in such a system), it abdicates in favour of the known laws of chemistry and physics (Sheldrake 1985).

The majority of scientifically trained minds would agree that the obvious way of explaining the effects of touching is in terms of physiology. Using this discipline, it is possible to ascertain that different areas of the body show different kinds of sensitivity. Some areas are more sensitive to light touch, others to pressure, heat or certain textures, etc. This is a zone-dependent qualitative sensitivity. Similarly, it is possible to show that a given area of the body is more or less sensitive to the same kind of touch — ie, a zone-dependent, quantitative sensitivity. Physiological descriptions of the effects of touch would initially be in terms of the characteristics of mechano-receptor type, function, locality, quantity, etc.

Furthermore, it could be demonstrated that different kinds of tactile experience perceived by different anatomical regions in the body will influence different areas of the central nervous system in different ways. Such stimuli would, for example, influence neuro-anatomical centres of co-ordination of posture and movement, protective reflexes and sexuality. This could all be demonstrated, at least in principle, using physiological measuring equipment.

The problem of ontological conversion

However, the difficulty with this model is that there are no clear ways of understanding exactly how a specific tactile event will be meaningfully interpreted by a person. This is firstly because the mechanism by which a neurological impulse becomes a feeling of, say, pleasure, remains a philosophical problem. Electrochemical neurological phenomena cannot be described in the same way as emotions. They are ontologically distinct. At this point the language of physiology again needs to abdicate in favour of another discipline — this time psychology. An added problem at this stage is the existence of a large selection of useful and interesting psychological models suggested by various subdisciplines of psychology. These competing models can coexist within psychology because their validity cannot be refuted using strict scientific criteria, since such criteria are located once more in a different discipline. It has simply become customary to describe physiological and psychological events in styles that are practically mutually exclusive.

The problem of infinite variables

There is a second problem with making a direct connection between physiological events and their meaning. In doing so it would be necessary to standardise the procedure of converting a measurable neurological event into an immeasurable psychological and emotional experience. Even if it were possible to bypass the philosophical impasse of ontological conversion and describe a system for translating neurological events into psychological language, the meaning of a touch to an individual is nevertheless a far subtler notion than is the mere stimulation of a postural reflex pattern. Similarly, one instance of an individual's experience of his or her sexuality is different from the mere experimental stimulation of sexual arousal. Sensations will mean different things to different people because each person is an individual. Meaning is biography-dependent in a manner that is infinitely complex and subtle. Because each person is unique, the predictive value of a hypothetical system of translation would be exceedingly poor. It is extremely unlikely that psychological events can ever become neurologically definable because the same psychologically definable events (such as my thought of tomorrow's weather and my wife's thought of tomorrow's weather) are certain to be represented by quite different neural configurations (Boorse 1976).

The physiological model allows us to explore only what is within the realms of physiology. These realms have distinct barriers when carefully scrutinised — with chemistry over the boundary at one end and psychology at the other. Physiological sciences can never give an adequate answer to the question 'what happens when you touch someone?' even when this is referring to manipulative touch. It can, however, contribute usefully to the answer. It is important to realise that the argument here is not that therapeutic touch-related physiological events are unable to help bring about, for example, feelings of drowsiness, well-being or the feeling of being cared for, but that they are not in themselves sufficient explanations of such feelings and cannot become so. In proportion as the nature of the patient's experience moves out of the realms of the biological (eg drowsiness) and verges on the subtle and conceptual (eg being valued or healed), so the value of the physiological explanation declines. The notion that manipulative touching does have non-physiological meaning capable of influencing health is of course the thesis of this book.

That physiological events are involved in healing both diseased tissues and persons feeling ill is not to be denied. An essential part of the analysis of the physiological explanation of a therapeutic touch is the concept that doing mechanical things to bodies has physiological effects. This notion, which obviously underpins much of medicine, is explored in more detail in the section on the physiological rationales of manual therapy.

Experiential explanations

Experience is the actual living through an event or events, and the effect upon the judgement or feelings produced by personal and direct impressions. It is usually taken to mean the conscious living through of such events (*ex* = out). However it is necessary also to take into account the unconscious since it is universally accepted that unconscious events form the iceberg of which the conscious mind is but the tip. The literature concerning itself with the effects of mental and emotional events on bodily processes will not be considered here. What is of concern is the nature of these events, and the nature of the language used to describe them — the everyday language of interpersonal communication.

As explained previously, physiological descriptions and language come to a dead end at the psychological end of their spectra. Therefore, it is pointless to ask a question such as 'why does holding/touching a baby in such and such a way make it feel valued?' and expect a fully adequate answer in physiological terms. This is firstly because there is no guarantee of locating any reproducible neural configuration typically representing being valued (the problem of infinite variables). Since repeatability is the hallmark of a scientific hypothesis, then such a unique finding is of little scientific value. Second, an experience of being valued (unconscious and instinctive in this case) is, as explained above, part of a different category of reality from a neural configuration (the problem of ontological conversion).

Allowing a wider context

If the question is posed without expecting an answer in terms of physiology, an answer may instead arise in terms of the meaning of a caress, rather than the physics of it. The criteria for such an answer would be observations concerning the use of holding itself within human relationships. It can be concluded that instinctive touching behaviour towards babies exists due to the biological 'rightness' of such behaviour. In the absence of this touching, infants would necessarily lack an adequate self-worth and self-confidence and this would mar their psychological and social development. The phenomenological explanation here is that holding a baby in this way *is* valuing it or loving it because that is how valuing or loving is enacted in the world. Indeed, it could be argued that the concepts of valuing and loving depend upon the existence of certain acts of touching for their full significance.

Taking this explanation further yields the notion that holding a baby close restores the wholeness or unity of what was until so recently one — mother and child. It is an expression of the desire to be at one with the child, and to satisfy the baby's need to be at one with its mother. Love as a generic term can be defined philosophically as the desire to merge with that which is loved. By this explanation the act of holding becomes an act of love, which necessarily includes the notion of valuing someone by touching them. Most patients feel this at some level, when being treated.

In adopting these types of phenomenological explanations, it is reasonable to talk about touch being used to show empathy, care, love, concern, desire, fear, insecurity, etc. Within these explanations reference is made to the way that touch is universally used in the whole context of observable psychological and anthropological behaviour and meaning.

For example, during a medical procedure, it might be observed that a patient's blood pressure falls while a nurse holds his hand. It is reasonable to argue that this occurred due to a reduction in the patient's anxiety created by his sense of shared vulnerability with the nurse. This may have reduced his own vulnerability, and enhanced his sense of self-worth (ie, a subconscious realisation that 'I am worth touching'). Self-worth enhances the sense of personal power, which in turn decreases fear and anxiety. This and other similar explanations are able quite legitimately to describe the effects of such nursing behaviour. It is not necessary to rely upon physiological theories of sympathetic nervous system tone reduction or endorphin release. These physiological effects are in any case probably best explained in terms of decreased anxiety rather than as end products of particular tactile stimulation. That is, the physiological effects derive from the psychodynamic events, not vice-versa.

Summary of the limits of physiology

As Western medical scientific thought has evolved it has become focused upon a peculiar and highly specialised aspect of humanity. The language of physiology has likewise become separated off from the range of normal language and so exclusive that it cannot embrace commonly used ideas related to interpersonal transactions. The specialisation necessary for physiological endeavour may well require a particular language, but in which case its use should be policed and it should be prevented from being used to describe events that take place partly or completely beyond its boundaries. Science itself is seductive and it is this quality that has led to the deploying of its language styles in contexts where they do not belong.

In the description of the human condition, physiological explanations are severely limited compared with psychological and philosophical ones. They may actually be misleading due to their having become over-emphasised and over-exposed. We may have become over-familiar with and over-reliant upon a small physiology section of a very large library of the human constitution.

The growth of phenomenology in medical theory

The philosopher Maurice Merleau-Ponty (1989) described the human body as being a 'primal element'. By this he meant that living human flesh can never be considered as if it were an inanimate object because it is that which allows us to experience inanimate objects. The body is both perceiver and perceived, actor and that which is acted upon. In an essential way the body *as it is lived* is unavailable for scrutiny because, for example, perceiving and doing are subjective phenomena. One can never really see the act of seeing. Only certain biochemical properties may therefore be disclosed to third parties, but never the body in the drama of its life (Leder 1990). The search for ways of describing the 'lived body' which are adequate enough to include the significance of human experience in both pathogenesis and healing has led to a surge of interest in phenomenological philosophy. This philosophy is seen as a way of rethinking medical language and is discussed further in Chapter 5.

The phenomenologist–medic Drew Leder argues that the material body as flesh, 'available' as anatomy and physiology, is merely an aspect of the lived body. In which case the scientific view should be placed within the first person experience, with the effect that the experiential domain would be liberated from its currently second-class citizenship. Because scientific strategies are specialised and uncommon ones, they should be reserved for their own, peculiar, third-person contexts. Instead, Leder says, we should recall the more common perspectives.

THE MIND AND THE BODY

The experiential and the physiological are aspects of the larger groups of mind and body (or soul and body). Inherent in modern scientific medical thought is the tendency not only to consider the two as essentially separate, but further, and paradoxically, to emphasise the body in matters of ill-health despite the concurrent necessity of locating the *self* in the mind as the observing agent. It is as if the mind and emotions are irrelevant in affairs of health, though over-qualified to theorise about it.

The reasons for this state of affairs having come about are complex. The situation has arisen against a backdrop of a decline in religio-mystical thought and practices, and the fall from favour of abstract and theosophical philosophy in the West. In addition, and inversely, material phenomena have become increasingly dominant as the focus of inductive scientific reasoning. All ancient religious philosophies included the idea that the soul was relevant where the development of ill-health was concerned, and provided the basis of a framework within which this relevance could be understood. (An example of such an all-embracing, ancient system of philosophy still in use today — hence an exception in this account — is traditional Chinese medical philosophy.) Because the soul and spirit were given so much prominence in everyday life, it was natural that they remained prominent in matters of ill-health and healing. (The existential profundity of severe and frequent infectious diseases probably contributed to this prominence.) As scientific thought developed, the void in the understanding of 'the constitution of man' left by the disappearance of theosophy was filled by the growth of materialism and with the familiar materialistic doctrines of human bodily constitution.

The extraordinary and glamorous achievements of technology have engulfed the mainstream health care professions exactly because the human body appears to be entirely located in this material world. It therefore subscribes to the kind of scrutiny at which modern science is so meticulously proficient.

Scientific enquiry with its emphasis on inductive reasoning and reproducible experiments has tended to drive out other varieties of enquiry such as the philosophico-psychological as a result of its own success and application. However, it is important to remember its limitations. It is only capable of operating in the observable, quantifiable, physical world. The extent of this reliance upon quantifiability in science culminates in one of its most important ideas; that scientific endeavour should be free of value and judgement, independent of human characteristics and of the beliefs and world-views of the scientist. In principle, scientists of different racial and cultural backgrounds ought to be able to work on the same projects in different parts of the world and come up with the same 'answers'.

Persons are not only 'scientific'

Persons, however, do hold and express beliefs, values, world-views, experiences, idiosyncrasies. They express sentiments and have feelings. They are emotional, irrational and unpredictable. Art in all its manifestations — from the pragmatic to the intellectual; painting, sculpture, dance, music, literature, education, morality, etc. — is testimony to that wealth of humanity that does *not* lend itself to scientific enquiry. If the subject of health care is a person, it necessarily follows that modern scientific methods operating at the physiological level only, will be inadequate to understand and deal with the person's health.

This conclusion is only valid if a further premise is also valid — that these psychological, emotional, social and spiritual aspects of a person are involved in health and wellness, illness and disease. All the evidence to date is in favour of this premise. There is no evidence that human beings are, in general, getting healthier mainly and specifically as a result of modern, scientific medical interventions. Disabling low back pain is a case in point. It is the cause of over a hundred million working days lost each year in the UK, and the most frequent symptom presenting to manual practitioners. Despite the increasing availability of treatment it continues to increase in prevalence (Frymoyer & Gordon 1989).

The denial of the psyche and the fate of psychosomatics

René Descartes is generally regarded as the originator of the divorce of mind from body, but the ancient Greeks also thought that a human being was in certain senses divisible. Plato's position is, roughly, that whereas the cosmos is dualistic in nature, being on the one hand abstract, spiritual, and intangible, and on the other hand material, corporeal, and tangible, human beings are tripartite (as is the Deity — hence the Christian doctrine of man as an image of the Deity). They are spiritual in essence, but exist in a corporeal realm and therefore have a material body. But the true self is, according to Plato, located in the soul, which must tackle the problems of being perpetually drawn between two polarities. Plato himself even complained that the medicine of his day neglected the soul in matters of healing.

Whereas in all mystical and religious traditions, human beings must strive to move from the material to the spiritual, emphasising the intellectual and the moral in order to move higher, modern scientific (and political) strategies emphasise material existence. The paradox is that the mind is put to brilliant use in mathematics, chemistry and physics as applied to the study of the body, but the study of the mind is denied the same political status as these disciplines (not least because it will not lie down and be observed whilst also doing the observing). Furthermore, Western man has become more unnatural, more unsensual, more dissociated and unaware of his body than ever before, in proportion as it has become the object of only materialistic, rather than affective exploration.

Plato's emphasis, aside from theistic doctrines, is to locate the self in the soul with particular emphasis on the mind. One should perfect one's outward activities so that these reflect a perfect spiritual world into which one thereby moves. All bodily activities were hence given explicit relational and symbolic significance. All ancient religious theosophies proposed a hierarchical organisation of man which began with the abstract and moved downward to gross bodily existence. Implicit in these doctrines are therefore causal and two-way relationships within the continuum of spirit–soul–body — or mind and body as it is usually described.

Descartes' contribution to the mind/body divorce was to locate the self in the abstract mind. He then used only certain philosophical strategies to understand what appeared to be objective to it — such as the body. He has not been noted for his concern with the exploration of the mind, or its betterment, despite having being a theist and a firm believer in the health-giving power of positive thought. It is not surprising that the emphasis of science has been on the material world because Descartes failed satisfactorily to demonstrate the relationship between the abstract mind and its material body. Furthermore, in promoting the study of the value-free corporeal world, because of its observability, he unwittingly discouraged further dialectic philosophy and also the belief of the essential integrality of mind and body. Without this emphasis the subject of health or illness would be located in the self, not merely the body. Psychology would have become as respectable as surgery, and psychosomatic medical theory would have become the norm.

However, not only did psychosomatic medicine not become the norm but psychology itself came to be considered as unscientific — pseudoscience at best. It is not so much that mental and emotional phenomena have so far eluded scientific enquiry, rather that they were excluded from it. There is no difficulty in regarding psychology as the 'science of the psyche' if it is recalled that the word 'science' simply means knowledge or knowing in general and not a particular type of knowing (just as 'art' is doing in general rather than a peculiar species of doing).

CONCLUSIONS

The question of psychologically significant manipulative touch

Mechano-physiological rationales for touching patients are adequate if practitioners agree to omit ideas about 'whole-person' healing and psychology from their discussions of the therapeutic encounter. At this stage in the proceedings, the question is not 'should manipulative practitioners always attend to the patient's psyche?', but rather 'under what circumstances can they avoid so doing?'.

Even if special psychological events always occur as a result of therapeutic touching, there will be occasions — perhaps many — when it will not be necessary to pay attention to these events. In the case of the head-cradling-cum-lateral fluctuation technique cited above, it seems reasonable that a psychological component is more likely to be significant, than, say, in a forearm muscle massage. This is because the head and face are much more associated with self-identity than is an arm. In addition and because of this, touching the head is a more intimate act. The nature of the psychological event triggered by the practitioner's touch — its emotional content — will depend partly upon which area of the body is touched.

Naturally it will also depend upon the character of the touching act. For example, to a patient, holding techniques feel different from moving techniques. The former feel like acts of 'being with', whereas the latter feel like acts of 'doing to'. Importantly, being with patients suggests human companionship (expressive touch), whereas doing things to them suggests an active/passive relationship more common when dealing with inanimate objects (procedural touch). Similarly, slow techniques invoke quite different psychological reactions from fast techniques; light touch from deep pressure; prolonged contact from staccato, and so on.

In these examples, the psychological impact of manual treatment depends upon anatomical and kinetic criteria. These are relatively predictable. However, the experience of each patient is unique and distinctive, a complex symphony of subconscious and conscious, past and present psychological and somatic issues encompassing healing, intimacy, physicality and being cared for. The psychological significance of manual therapy remains a rich and unexplored field for research.

What manipulative practitioners say they do

It is probably accurate to say that osteopaths, chiropractors, physiotherapists and other manual practitioners believe that they are able to cause changes in the flesh of their patients by manipulating it. There will be some practitioners who will object to the implied dualism of this statement. They would counter that they treat people rather than manipulate flesh. Some of the implications of this humanistic or holistic attitude to therapy are explored later in this book. However, it is useful to employ such terminology in order to help clarify the physiological viewpoint. Furthermore, since it is unlikely that this statement will be passionately opposed by the majority of practitioners, and if the available literature describes only physiological rationales for manual therapy, then manipulating flesh is currently the more accurate term.

A variety of different manipulative techniques are described in the literature and there is diverse opinion on under what conditions (ie dysfunctional states of tissue) certain techniques should be used. There are also descriptions of how best to use these techniques for the different conditions. Anyone who has been a patient of more than one practitioner will know that no two of them do exactly the same thing — even when presented with similar conditions. This is partly explained by the expressive peculiarities of the individual practitioner; how they express themselves through movement. In addition it is recognised within the professions that the different approaches to patient care adopted by different practitioners are a result of:

- the existence of a variety of therapeutic models and approaches to manual therapy which are apparently applicable to similar presenting conditions
- different techniques and ways of working within these models — for example, 'functionally', or 'structurally' (analogous to homoeopathic and allopathic)
- practitioners' choice in utilising these models, depending on educational experiences and attitudes.

It is clear that manual practitioners touch their patients in many different ways. These differences are partly determined by intellectual conceptions of how change is caused to occur in tissues according to philosophical, mechanical and physiological principles, and partly by the individual expressive behaviour and attitudes of each practitioner. Psychological theories explaining the results of manipulation are largely absent from the literature, as is the notion of practitioners' character-dependent expressive touch.

Rationales are disputed

Although it is recognised within the professions that there are different practical and theoretical ways of being a manipulative practitioner, these different approaches are sometimes frowned upon. It is not accepted by all members of the osteopathic profession for example that there is a clear and distinct definition of osteopathy — let alone what that definition might amount to. There is considerable disagreement about what kind of a theory would be useful and appropriate — how much philosophy, physiology, mechanics and psychology would be incorporated into it, and what activities are properly 'osteopathic' rather than belonging to some other discipline. In particular, there is disagreement over the extent to which osteopaths should adhere to the writings of their founder A T Still, or to the words of those practitioners to whom the wisdom has been personally handed down through the ages. Should these writings be closely followed, or should osteopaths continually develop theories in relation to the concepts and assumptions which underlie the practice of health care in general and manual medicine in particular? This and other controversies within theoretical osteopathy are divisive, but also potentially creative.

There is somewhat less dissent in the chiropractic profession, and little amongst physiotherapists. In the case of the former this is probably because of the arguably more focused and single-minded development of theoretical chiropractic (see, for example, Haldeman 1992). Physiotherapy has usually considered itself an integral part of medicine and has not felt the need to define itself as being unique and distinct from medicine in general, as have the other two professions.

In the osteopathic profession, the phrases 'osteopathy is that which is practised by osteopaths', and more enigmatically 'osteopathy is that which A T Still had in mind when he coined the phrase' are often heard. This is not because it pleases members of the profession to assume ownership of mysterious skills, but because simple definitions have not emerged, since they would not suit the practice of osteopathy. In a society where there is an observable return to 'whole person' attitudes towards health care, and where linear, bioreductionist theories and attitudes have passed their historical peak, it would be surprising if such a simple definition had arisen and been adhered to. The ambiguity within this body of theoretical manipulative medicine lends credence to a thesis arguing the case for psychologically significant touch.

What manipulative practitioners actually do

The following playful paragraph is also intended to make the serious point that the way in which manipulative therapy is regarded may be blinkered. This has been brought about by the near complete absorption of manipulative therapy into the belly of modern medicine. Its true place may actually be in the much broader context of healing.

'What seems to happen within the practice of manual medicine is that two persons form a relationship with certain characteristics. One person, who usually wears a white coat, stays in the same building all

week and is paid by the other. The other has to take nearly all her clothes off after a brief chat, and then is touched a lot — pushed, pulled, held, rubbed, rocked, kneaded. This involves about the same amount of physical contact as a wrestling match or heavy petting — although it is not overtly violent or erotic. Sometimes there is just a light touch of one or two areas. The whole encounter lasts about half an hour or more, and many such visits may occur.' (anon.)

This decontextualised description of the contract highlights ambiguities and reminds one of the range of possibilities when considering a theory for such an interaction. The description in the previous paragraph deliberately emphasises the intimate nature of the encounter, the possible erotic or violent connotations, and the obvious power discrepancy between the practitioner and the patient (one acting upon, the other being acted upon; one lying down, the other standing or sitting; one relinquishing control of her body over to the other). And yet this is a health care practitioner skilled in bodily manipulation 'treating'a patient — to use a safe, sterile, medicalised description.

What really goes on? How might we describe it? Are we to accept simple mechanical theories of reordering joint and muscle symmetry, torsion and balance, or neurophysiological theories of viscero-somatic reflex, segmental dysfunction or fluid dynamics? Should we also theorise in terms of psychosomatics, emotional blocking, body armouring and postural symbology?

It is a fact that the manipulative professions have so far involved themselves very little with psychosomatic or whole-person medicine because the majority of their theories remain articulated in bio-reductionistic terminology. Without a fundamental change in terminology and in the context in which they place their work, they will remain unable to develop fuller, adequate explanations of their art. Indeed, the danger is that they will try to refine, complete and perfect a fundamentally deficient, somewhat tautological and self-limiting thesis. If this is the case any aspirations to holism or effective psychosomatics will be doomed.

The present understanding of the effect of the manual therapy encounter is not merely in need of details to fill in the gaps — rather it is in need of a shift in attitude; from this will spring a different kind of understanding.

SUMMARY OF MAIN POINTS

This chapter has:

1. introduced the notion of two types of touch, the technical and expressive, together with examples, and suggested that both types are important in clinical practice
2. criticised an exclusively physiological approach to understanding human beings and therapeutic touching
3. suggested that it is reasonable to use non-scientific language to describe persons and certain interpersonal health care encounters
4. introduced the notion of psychologically significant touch, with a brief historical account of interest in the psyche
5. asserted that the majority of manual practitioners use only physiological descriptions of their work, many of which are controversial within the professions
6. concluded with the challenge to theoretical manual therapy to step back and take a wider theoretical view of its subject matter.

This book goes on to examine some of the theories currently under the umbrella of manual therapy, with particular reference to the act of touching. The reader will find little reinterpretation of the already widely interpreted principles given by present and past masters of the professions. This is not because they are inadequate, but because they are based upon further assumptions, in need of philosophical exploration for which there is no space in this text. Nor is there scope fully to describe all the theoretical physiological and mechanical rationales put forward to underpin manual therapy in general (further reading is suggested). The book summarises the most important and influential ideas, questions and assumptions. More importantly, it goes on to explore those further subjects which suggest themselves sufficiently strongly as being relevant to the work of manual therapy, that they cannot help but become incorporated into its body of knowledge.

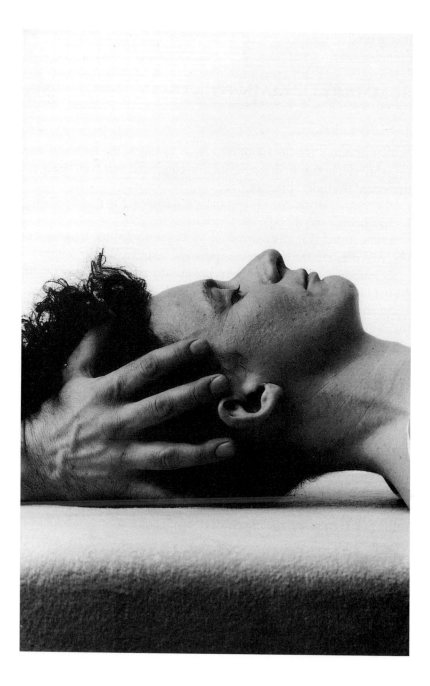

REFERENCES

Boorse C 1976 What a theory of mental health should be. Journal for the Theory of Social Behaviour 6(1): 61–84

Brody H 1992 The healer's power. Yale University Press (p 7)

Frymoyer J W, Gordon S L 1989 Research perspectives in low back pain. Spine 14: 1384–1390

Haldeman S (ed) 1992 Principles and practice of chiropractic, 2nd edn. Appleton & Lange, Connecticut

Leder D 1990 The absent body. University of Chicago Press, Chicago

Merleau-Ponty M 1989 Phenomenology of perception. Routledge & Kegan Paul, London

Sheldrake R 1985 A new science of life: the hypothesis of formative causation. Anthony Blond, London, chs 1 & 2

2

Is manual therapy only technology and procedure?

Psychological implications of mechanical and physiological rationales

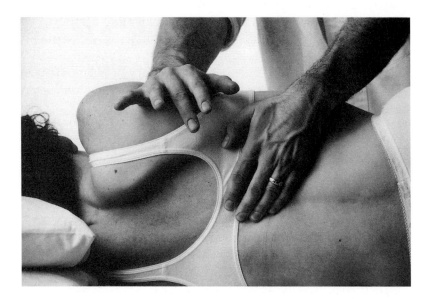

Introduction

The manipulative professions have been eager to gain acceptance by orthodox, Western, medicine. They have striven to perceive themselves as rooted in it by taking pains to demonstrate the efficacy of their art in the common language of mechanics and physiology.

The previous chapter claimed that virtually all available explanations underlying manual therapy are mechanical and physiological in nature. It was asserted that since physiological terminology may be inadequate to make sense of emotional and experiential events, it failed to do justice to these aspects of treatment. However, since most research and literature concerning psychosomatics are in terms of neuroendocrine events, and because physiology is the accepted language of medicine, it is necessary to explore how the psychological significance of manual therapy may emerge from a consideration of conventional theory.

The objectives of this chapter are:

- to describe the basis upon which all physiological theories underlying manual therapy depend
- to discover the questions begged by these theories
- to ascertain whether these questions are those which necessitate a broadening of theoretical manual medicine in the direction of psychological subjects.

UNORTHODOX MANUAL THERAPY AND SUBTLE ENERGY THEORY

Within the theoretical framework of the major schools of manual therapy — chiropractic, osteopathy and manipulative physiotherapy — and other therapies relying upon massage-type processes, are references to models of health and illness of a psychosomatic nature. Such references are probably not given their just exposure. Some of them are explicit in the literature, whilst others are implied by the use of certain philosophical models or concepts.

To begin with, it should be pointed out that there are certain schools of manual therapy that do not propose a physiological basis for understanding treatment processes. In these schools, if the physiological is included, it is done so after the more important events have occurred — and *because* they have occurred. Examples of such disciplines are shiatsu, therapeutic touch, polarity therapy, reiki, the various schools of 'laying on of hands', and other examples of 'energetic' healing.

Instead, models are proposed, all of which include the notion of energy fields interacting causally with physiological processes. It is to these fields of energy that practitioners direct their therapeutic attention. An interesting but little-recognised fact is that these energetic theories of the human constitution are derived from both Eastern (Indian, Chinese), Middle Eastern (Persian) and Western (Greek) traditional theosophy. They include explanations of the nature of that relation between the human spirit and the coarse matter of the body. In their original form, these writings trace energy and form from spirit down through hierarchically arranged 'subtle bodies' — including the emotional — culminating in the coarse matter of physical body. It is from these subtle subsistencies that the notion of a field of energy is descended.

Crucially, both acupuncture (a medical discipline more than 3000 years old) and homoeopathy address themselves specifically to these subtle energetics, which are judged capable of influencing physiological processes in the body. It is explicit in these disciplines that emotional and psychological energy influence, and are influenced by, energetic determinants of bodily form and function. This is why acupuncture and homoeopathy include concepts of emotional and psychological health care within their theoretical frameworks.

Many manual practitioners, especially massage therapists and those less orthodox disciplines cited above, adhere to field theory and notions of energy transfer between practitioners and patients. In doing so, these practitioners are bound to consider emotional issues in their concepts of health care, and they hold that emotional and psychological phenomena are influenced by their work.

Whilst it is true that there exist writings by both chiropractors and osteopaths that include subtle-body theory in various forms, nevertheless within these professions this appears to be very much a minority approach. The founders of both osteopathy (Andrew Still) and chiropractic (Daniel Palmer) were vitalists, who believed that life force permeated and flowed through human beings. It was the practitioner's job to remove mechanical impediments to that flow. A patient's psychological ill-health was thus just as capable of being influenced by treatment as bodily ill-health was, because both were regarded as functions of vitality, frustrated by mechanical and other environmental events.

Had history taken a different course, and not resulted in a suppression of these more abstract systems of philosophy, then manual therapy and orthodox medicine would have naturally embraced emotional medicine.

THE BASIC ASSUMPTIONS OF MANUAL MEDICINE: PREMISES ONE AND TWO

The essential premise of manual medicine is very straightforward: it is necessary that, in doing what appear to be mechanical things to their patients, manual practitioners expect beneficial physiological results to take place. This expectation of effects which are both specific and good rests upon the notion of a more or less predictable relationship between the mechanical and the physiological. This premise will be referred to as premise one.

A second premise fundamental to all medicine including the manual therapies is that there are inherent healing, repair and regulatory mechanisms constantly operating; for example, acute inflammation and resolution, or an immune response to and resolution of a systemic infection. The activities of modern Western medicine have tended to obscure inherent healing because their interventions commonly take place when such self-healing systems appear all but spent. However, no system of theoretical medicine denies the supremacy of such a

---

Box 2.1   Basic assumptions of manual medicine

- Premise one: practitioners' manual acts on patients' bodies cause beneficial physiological effects.
- Premise two: there are inherent self-repair, self-healing and self-regulatory mechanisms at work in the body.

homeostatic or more properly 'homeodynamic' principle. This premise will be referred to as premise two.

These two concepts, seemingly obvious, are in need of further elaboration because upon them are based the entire repertoires of manual practitioners of virtually all kinds.

Physiologically significant mechanics: premise one in detail

1. The dynamic physical organisation of an area of the body — in the broadest sense — for example the head, can be regarded in terms of kinetic phenomena such as patterns of:
— bony and other joint movements
— intra-tissue and inter-tissue movements, pressures and tensions
— fluid movement characteristics
— fluctuations in tissue motility and elasticity
— positional variations over time, and so on.

2. These kinetic phenomena must logically operate within certain limitations imposed by various biological norms. This is in order that the different subsystems within the head might operate properly together in a healthy and adaptable way.

3. These kinetic[1] effects are clearly the outer manifestations or representations of an extremely complex interdependent and integrated system of inner physiological and biochemical phenomena.

4. It is reasonable to assume that the relationships existing between the inner and the outer events will be orderly and predictable, since it is unreasonable to expect such relationships to express chaos.

5. At least some of the outer mechanical phenomena would be detectable by palpation and capable of being influenced by manipulation.

6. Therefore, manual therapy reasons that the inner manifestations can be investigated by touching their outer representations.

7. For manual treatment to be physiologically significant, the inner physiological phenomena and the outer mechanical ones must be to some extent causally reversible or equivalent. That is, certain mechanical events must be able to influence certain physiological ones, and not merely vice versa. That this is the case is well accepted and illustrated by a consideration of the quantity, type, location and effects of

stimulation of mechanoreceptors. It is also illustrated by research into the effects of, for example, massage and exercise. Human tissue reacts to its mechanical environment in an orderly and organised way.

8. In the case of disordered functioning of any of these outer, physical phenomena (listed in 1. above), and therefore of their physiological equivalents, and the palpatory detection thereof, it is theoretically possible to reorder function. This is achieved by imposing forces, or boundaries, movements, pressure, negative pressure, etc., upon the body in specific and highly organised ways in order to influence positively the systems within. That is, help to restore health.

Important concepts

In summary, because in the body physiological events give rise to mechanical ones, which further cyclically influence the physiological systems, it is reasonable to argue that active forces from outside the body applied to it will cause physiologically significant mechanical events. If such forces from without were not physiologically significant, then this would be equivalent to the claim that the human body does not perceive and respond to its mechanical environment — which is clearly not the case.

It is true that the notion of mechanical events causing physiological ones is not a novel one — a swift blow to the head with a rosewood cosh, to use an unsubtle example, would quickly remind one of this. It is well known that physiological/biochemical activity within tissue is highly organised, but what is in need of emphasis is that *the outer, palpable kinetic and mechanical phenomena are as numerous, peculiar, highly organised and integrated as those inner physiological ones that they express.* This is because the relationship between the mechanical and the physiological is an organised (that is, predictable, orderly and normative) one.

Therefore, applying orderly manual treatment will influence physiological processes in a similarly predictable way.

A claimed knowledge of the normal (healthy) and abnormal (unhealthy) features of palpably detectable human physicokinetic phenomena could be considered peculiar to sophisticated and highly developed schools of manual medicine.

Premise one includes all specific theories available in the literature based on the physiological effects of mechanical therapy. Since the latter are too numerous they will not be explored piecemeal. Premise one can be regarded as a sufficient rationale for manual therapy. It demonstrates why touching patients may be used:

1. to perceive and receive meaningful tactile information
2. to conceive of and formulate judgements concerning the significance of such information
3. to administer manual techniques, depending upon judgements formulated.

However, it remains to be determined:

1. which kinds of manual event are physiologically significant
2. the degree to which manual events are physiologically significant
3. in what ways they are significant — that is, what are the physiological effects?

All this in turn depends upon the substance of the relationship between the mechanical and the physiological, especially the degree to which the mechanical expression of physiological events is reversible. It also depends upon an understanding of the organisational features of the mechanical environment of the body. Further aspects of this relationship are explored in the section on systems (p 51).

Psychological implications of premise one

Premise one argues that doing mechanical things to people's bodies can have beneficial physiological effects. This is so long as such acts are based upon an understanding of the mutually interactive nature of the relationship between physiology and mechanics. In order to claim that the same treatments are also psychologically significant, it is necessary to show either:

A. that there is a further mutually interactive relationship between the psychological and physiological, or/and

B. that the patient's perception of being touched — whether conscious or unconscious — has psychological effects prior to or regardless of any physiological ones directly generated by touching.

There are three basic views of mental events:

1. Mental events are electrochemical ones. That is, the mind is nothing more than brain tissue.
2. Mental events are of a hierarchically different order of reality than electrochemistry, and are expressed through it.
3. The two are not causally related, but are different expressions of the same reality; they are epiphenomena.

A. The notion that there is a mutually interactive relationship between the psychological and physiological

It should be pointed out that this is an extremely difficult area, and there is little agreement among philosophers. However, it makes no difference to this analysis whether mental events are considered as abstract or as electrochemical in nature. If they are *nothing but* electrochemical phenomena (which is the popular view though decreasingly so), then they are essentially physiological anyway. In which case the potency of manual therapy as a psychologically significant event is shown by premise one and its conditions. The extent of this potency and the kinds of psychological effect expected of manual therapy would then simply be a matter for clinical reasoning and research.

If psychological events (whether or not these are abstract or corporeal) are believed to *give rise* to physiological ones, then this can be regarded as an extension of premise one. In which case it would be reasonable to postulate that the outer physiological phenomena are as numerous, peculiar and highly organised as those psychological ones that they express. This is, again, because the relationship between the two is predictable, orderly and normative.

In the case of non-corporeal models of mentation, there still would have to exist the capacity for organised perception and response to physiological/mechanical events else there would be no feedback and integration between the two realms. It is noteworthy that the 'esoteric' philosophical systems giving rise to such models insist on care and orderly cultivation of the body and bodily habits, because this is seen as the prerequisite to soul culture. For example, Pythagoras' system of training especially emphasised care and attention of the body. Where the body is believed to be a vehicle through which the soul expresses itself, then alteration of the body will result in a change in the degree and quality of expressibility of the soul. Similarly, in the phenomenological view of life as 'embodied', then manual therapy will alter the possibilities for embodiment.

If mental and physiological events are epiphenomena then, since they reflect one another, the former would change along with the latter. In which case premise one again applies.

The conclusion is that, using premise one as a base for investigation, manual therapy is capable not merely of being strongly psychologically significant but also possibly psychotherapeutic. This is especially so in proportion as causation operates freely from the physiological to the psychological. Again, as at the conclusion of premise one in detail, the degree to which psychologically significant physiological mechanisms are capable of being influenced by therapeutic touch remains to be demonstrated. Indeed, which ones may so be influenced? These questions can only be resolved by open-minded and ethical clinical research.

B. The notion that *a patient's* perception *of being touched has central psychological effects prior to or regardless of any local physiological ones directly generated by touching*

The foregoing conclusion concerning the relationship between the physiological and psychological is based upon an ordered sequence of events whereby one becomes, or expresses, the other. However, this is a fairly limited and mechanical view of events. A further area for investigation is whether or not the perception of touch events triggers characteristic and unique psychological memories, feelings and other mental phenomena in each person, due to each's peculiar history. The evidence presented in this book strongly suggests that this is so. Such phenomena would be capable of participating significantly in the arousal of both positive and negative physiological responses pertinent to manual therapy.

This exploration of premise one has shown that the accepted philosophical underpinning of manual therapy's physiological effects also provides for psychological effects (A above). It does not include the notion of psychological effects being caused according to B above.

If the evidence for B occurring is convincing, which this book proposes, then the potential for psychological effects to occur during manual therapy is increased considerably.

Self-preservation and self-persistence concepts: premise two in detail

It is uncommon for the notion of inherent self-healing to be emphasised in orthodox medical textbooks. This is partly because it is taken for granted to the extent that it remains unnoticed, and partly because medical intervention often illustrates the view that the body-machine is being fixed rather than being aided in its own healing. But the reliance on self-healing is responsible for the most common medical procedure in general practice — masterly non-intervention *pauses* (in the case, for example, of the vast majority of self-limiting infective episodes). The most orthodox form of manual therapy, manipulative physiotherapy, likewise relies upon the concept of inherent self-healing as much as less orthodox disciplines. *(it's form of "masterly non-intervention")?*

By contrast, theoretical chiropractic and osteopathy constantly refer to notions of self-healing or the body's 'innate intelligence' as a central theme around which their manual interventions are organised. Both these disciplines have always laid emphasis on the examination of their philosophical roots, because they have been conscious of a need to carve a permanent place for themselves in health care — a place both unique and reasonable. It is this obsession with philosophical concepts that has led to considerable exposure of the innate intelligence principle. However, it is important to remember that this principle is vital to all systems of healing from the most to the least orthodox.

'*The business of the doctor is to distract the patient whilst nature does the healing.*' (anon.)

Manual therapeutics, then, rely upon the kinetic or mechanical analogue of homeostatic self-healing — 'homeokinesis'. Kinetic or mechanical properties which are dysfunctional or which reflect or represent underlying dysfunctional physiological states will tend to move towards a healthy state. If they do not, it must be because normal adaptability is disrupted or environmental changes have overcome the body's capacity for self-maintenance (Martinke 1991).

The interventions of manual medicine are said to enhance, enable or restore those physiologico-kinetic processes that represent inherent tendencies towards health. Emphasis is often on allowing self-righting processes to occur, rather than on imposing new ones. Some manual practitioners insist that they do not actually do anything except provide, using touch, bodily environmental conditions that facilitate such self-righting processes.

It is partly because orthodox medicine concentrates so much upon serious disease warranting radical intervention and invasive techniques, that the notion of self-healing is not emphasised. Noticeably, orthodox medicine specialises very much in cases where normal adaptability is markedly disrupted. Attention paid to self-healing is therefore minor compared with that paid to frank intervention.

Manual practitioners may be more able to indulge themselves in self-healing phenomena at their level of intervention because such intervention is relatively minimal. Processes of self-regulation and the body's capacity for self-maintenance may be more viable, conspicuous and accessible to manual practitioners. This is because the disruption of function and regulation is less severe in their patients. Accordingly, it is likely that manual practitioners' claim that they are working with and assisting the body's self-healing, self-regulatory processes is not so much a matter of differing philosophy as it is a matter of emphasis.

Psychological implications of premise two

If the view of a human being is as a physicochemical machine, then processes of self-regulation, defence and repair, adaptation to environmental demand, and self-replication, would be analogous only to the most elaborate artificial instrumentation (eg a computer). But because such artificial processes have not been created and are not understood except in outline, then there is in reality no analogy. If one is used, therefore, it probably perpetuates an unhelpful myth (Sheldrake 1985).

Defence and repair are aspects of self-preservation, which is necessary in order that the organism might persist. Persistence, maintained only partly by defence and repair processes, should be viewed as an attribute firstly of human beings, not merely of human bodies. This is because the efficiency of defence and repair processes is capable of *the person is persisting not the body*

considerable modification by psychological and emotional events.[2] Such events do not lend themselves to purely mechanistic descriptions. The notion of the *body's* capacity to defend and repair itself is therefore misleading unless qualified by reference to those processes sufficiently mechanical to be predicable only of the body, and not of the person (if indeed, the two can ever be separated). The loss of the personal context is a false device.

Self-regulatory processes, likewise, are predicated of the body, and none would doubt their existence. But here too, a similar objection could be raised — that because self-regulatory processes are capable of modification by emotional events, then self-regulation does not lend itself to purely mechanical description. It is therefore more correctly predicated of persons, not bodies. Again, purely *bodily* self-regulation must only refer to those processes sufficiently mechanical in nature to be considered as only bodily processes. But in reality these are part of a greater personal system.

The claim fully to understand a complicated homeostatic phenomenon without a parallel claim to know its context and initiation is inadequate. This is especially so when the initiating causes are emotional or symbolic ones. The wealth of research literature concerning the placebo effect alone demonstrates the extraordinary influence of mental events upon processes of self-regulation and healing (Roberts 1993).

It is simply inaccurate, therefore, to use the term 'mechanisms' when describing human self-regulation, self-defence and self-repair processes in their entirety, as much as it is inaccurate to refer to a person as a body. The human attribute of self-persistence renders those processes contributing to it as being teleological. Such processes operate in order that the human being as a whole might persist, and they minister to the minute-to-minute and year-to-year plans and aims of each purposive human life.

This brief consideration of premise two, then, should enlarge the context in which self-regulatory and self-healing processes are placed. Such processes are part of each *person's* means and are subject to the forces of emotion.

Self-expression and self-assertion too, even if these are merely instinctive and not rationalised in the mind, can be seen to be even more goal-centred than self-preservation. Self-expression and self-assertion give rise to much physiological and mechanical bodily activity. It is essential, then, that such activity is seen as *embodied life* together with meanings, feelings and purposes, and not merely as physiological clockwork.

THE SYSTEMS VIEW AND INTEGRATED FUNCTIONING

All manual practitioners pay at least lip service to the concept of 'integrated functioning' of the human body. For example, if a part of the body appears to be malfunctioning then:

- that part will affect the entire body economy to some extent
- the distinctive functioning of the entire body will affect the malfunctioning part in certain ways, and might have contributed to its malfunction
- the malfunctioning part may influence or be influenced by one or more other areas remote from it.

The concept is useful both for laying emphasis on the necessity for addressing the therapeutic aim to the entire body, and for implicating remote areas of the body in cases of local disorder. The 'whole is more than the sum of the parts' is the familiar cliché in need of interpretation.

What the concept is trying to convey is that there is something else besides the mere summation of body parts which goes to make up the whole body. According to the systems view, that something is organisation. The systems view of the body conforms particularly well to that view taken by manual therapists, and especially by osteopaths. Because systems theory in its 'pure' form has long been a respected model for understanding organisations, its application to manual therapy theory is worthy of note. The acceptance of systems theory into manual therapy theory also entails the acceptance of certain psychological implications which are outlined in the next section. Relevant aspects of the theory are considered below.

The word 'system' (rather than 'part' or 'structure') is used in the manner suggested by Angyal in his chapter 'A Logic of Systems' (Angyal 1981). A knowledge of this work is not necessary fully to understand or appreciate the argument. However, to clarify, the use of 'system' serves to emphasise that any major part (system) of the body — for example the head and neck, the upper limb complex, the trunk, etc — is:

bodily system is
- part of a greater whole or suprasystem
- composed of subsystems which are inter-related such that each can be fully understood only in terms of the arrangement–relationships which exist between them, and between them and their suprasystem. They cannot be understood purely in terms of their composition. *as above, so below; getting to know the mind of God*

The nature of the arrangements between the systems, subsystems, and suprasystems is the essential concept. It should always be given at least as much importance as an analysis of the nature and characteristics of the parts themselves.

Premise one stated that physiological activity is presented to manual practitioners in the form of patterns of palpable, kinetic events. Patterns are qualities which are organisational in nature. Manual practitioners' understanding of the organisational features of the mechanical environment of the body ought, therefore, to be considerable, and at the forefront of their clinical thought processes. The following attributes of a system are drawn from Angyal (1981).

The nature of systems

1. Classes of tissues versus systems of tissues

Body 'systems', according to the usual use of the word, are defined by virtue of the similar features of their members, for example, morphological characteristics (histology) or function. These are obviously related. In this way different members of the system can be identified. Only two members of this kind of system need be identified in order that the system should exist, because similarity is the only attribute. In fact, similarity between two structures is evidence of a *relation*, not a true *system* at all. A true system, by contrast, is organisational in nature, and members participate in it by virtue of their positional value in the whole system, not by any inherent quality.

For example, a vein and the connective or muscular tissue proximal to it participate in a true system because of their positional relationships. However, they are members of separate orthodox systems by virtue of their different inherent qualities. The inherent qualities are just that — they are qualities of the members, and not of the system itself. Positional relationships, however, are qualities of the true system. In fact, the orthodox system is not so much a system as a *class of tissues*. The orthodox use of system is therefore something of a misnomer unless explicit reference is made to organisational features — which is unusual.

The skeletal 'system' simply allows us to identify tissue as skeletal. The muscular 'system' allows us to identify tissue as muscular. If one asks 'what kind of a system is the muscular system?', the answer is 'one consisting of muscular tissue, causing movement of the body'. But 'muscular system' denotes a system of muscles. It ought to point to the notion of organisation. However, the usual use of the word is mere labelling, rather than emphasising the concept of systemic organisation. Schools of physical medicine have certainly discovered the subtleties of muscle organisation but this is not what is generally implied by the term 'muscular system'. Furthermore, such discoveries have largely excluded the relationships between muscular and other tissue. The word system has been used instead mainly to draw attention to the differences between tissues. It has been used as a tool for categorising tissue. Little useful information has therefore been allowed to emerge concerning relationships between tissues.

The colon, for example, in the ordinary way of thinking, is not considered part of the alimentary system by virtue of its position in the abdomen (which is highly variable anyway). Rather, it is because it is a hollow viscus, comparable histologically and functionally with, and continuous with the ileum above and the rectum below. It is true the colon tends to occupy a species-typical space in the abdominal cavity, but this position is not the essential feature that identifies it as alimentary (rather than reproductive, for example) in nature. Rather, then, the usual meaning of the word 'system' in medical textbooks concerns functionally similar components. The cardiovascular system consists of the heart and blood vessels, the alimentary system consists of a tube from mouth to anus with associated glandular tissue, the neurological system consists of the brain, spinal cord and peripheral nerves, and so on.

The usual anatomical habit of classing similar tissues together as members of a system in order to emphasise common physiological properties has resulted in an over-emphasis on categorisation of groups of tissue. This has rendered the categories somehow more distinct and significant than they really are. It has mislaid the organisational features denoted by the word 'system'. If there is an attitude of over-specialisation with which each such class of tissue has been regarded, then this emphasis upon tissue property is probably responsible.

To predicate true systemic organisation of a set of tissues where there may in fact be little, is to prevent the observation of how true bodily systems operate by drawing the attention away from more subtle organisational features of body regions.

It is difficult to see the systemic organisation of, say, the shoulder, when it is said to be composed of elements of the skeletal, muscular, fascial, nervous, vascular, and perhaps other systems. There is no word left to describe the *system* of the shoulder, as the word has been imprecisely appropriated. This is not to say that the musculoskeletal system does not display true systemic characteristics. Rather, it is to emphasise that the usual use of 'system' tends to veil the perception of the organisational significance of a whole area composed of many different types of tissue.

2. Dimension

The term 'muscular system', therefore, should draw attention to the dimensional characteristics of muscle tissue organisation. However, as stated above, it is usually used to draw attention to muscle tissue as distinct from other kinds. The role of dimension in an orthodox system is only to make its members distinct from each other. The dimension itself does not tend to participate in the system. The true system, however, is essentially dimensional in nature — it is a *dimensional domain*. The dimensions themselves give rise to the system's characteristic features because they are basic to geographical organisation. In emphasising the dimensional domain, the relationships between, say, left psoas major and descending colon could be worked out. These structures participate in the *system of the abdomen,* a true system. By usual reckoning such structures are members of separate systems and are explicitly unrelated.

3. *Contextual connection*

Members of an orthodox system participate in it by means of a more direct connection than do members of the true system — the connection requires no mediator. For example, the ascending and descending colon require reference to nothing else in order to make the connection between them as members of the alimentary system. This is because the relationship between them is only in terms of their similar, inherent quality. Likewise, the relation between gluteus medius and psoas major is that they are muscles. However, in the true system, members may not be significantly related to each other except with reference to the whole. To regard the abdomen, pelvis and lower extremities as subsystems of a suprasystem provides for a more complete understanding, for example, of the relationship between psoas major and gluteus medius, between psoas major and the colon, or even adductor longus and the vagina.

Likewise, the term 'the system of the neck and trunk' implies an organised zone comprising different tissues whose anatomical arrangements are physiologically significant, and not merely identifiable. It is not possible to witness the significance of the relationship between rectus abdominus and C5 facet joints except from a systemic viewpoint whereby prolonged hypertonia of the former may give rise to adaptive extension of the latter. Without the whole context the significant relationship between these structures remains undetected. The connection between such structures requires a detailed knowledge at least of the entire system(s) of the head, neck, thorax and abdomen. In this way one may fully understand the contribution they and other members make to the whole. Their interconnections are mechanical and physiological organisational relationships inherent in detailed anatomy.

In what system does the urinary bladder participate? The urinary system? Such an answer stifles inquiry. The bladder participates in the system of the sex-specific, abdomino-pelvis together with muscular, neurological and psychological regulating influences, and the influences of further, nearby viscera.

Physiologically significant organisation

The essential feature of the true system, then, is that it predicates profound organisational significance of the body, over and above, and in addition to, the properties of its different tissues. It is of course true that orthodox systems do predicate organisational significance of their members, but usually only of members of the same functionally related tissue. For example, there is significance in the positions of the cerebellum and basal ganglia, with respect to each other and with respect to the whole central nervous system, but this is inside, as it were, the feature of tissue similarity. It is nervous tissue that is being considered.

The relationships between and within suprasystems, systems, and subsystems can be biochemical, physiological (neurological, vascular, etc), mechanical/kinetic, psychological or symbolic. But it is how the subsystems are related in terms of mechanical forces that is the most immediately important aspect of the relationship. Adding premise one (the physiological significance of mechanics) to systemic organisation serves to emphasise the physiological relationships between the subsystems. Although this includes those physiological relationships not resulting from position (hormonal influences, for example), it is the significance of position that is emphasised.

For example, the participation of the colon in the true system of the abdomen is by virtue of its position relative to all other abdominal structures (as well as some pelvic and thoracic ones). This allows for the susceptibility of the colon to physiologically significant influence by these structures and vice versa.

It is of course well recognised that orthodox systems are inter-related physiologically. For example, the cardiovascular with the neurological, and both of these with all other systems. But in the main, those relationships between different tissues not directly related to the function or purpose of each system — the inter-tissue organisational significance — are not usually considered unless gross pathology occurs. This is because orthodox medicine is geared to 'end-stage' medicine, to frank pathology. In which case, the effects of one tissue on another by virtue of their position are far from subtle (for example, the presence of a pathological fissure in Crohn's disease, connecting the colon with other peritoneal structures).

[handwritten margin notes at top:] inconsistency - Milton "I love pathology"? Trager Ist. "We do not treat in Trager Approach"

[handwritten notes above first paragraph:] Milton was pathologically oriented - there is so much more that can happen when we recognize that treatment does not interfere fixing or pathology

For manual practitioners, the inter-tissue organisational significance is both apparent and relevant at all times, and not merely in cases of gross pathology. In the absence of such pathology, manual practitioners need to justify their concern with the positional value of tissues and kinetic/mechanical considerations. Justification is to be found in premise one which establishes such considerations as being consistently physiologically significant.

Contrasting attitudes

What emerges from this distinction is that, in orthodox thought, the body is analysed in terms of types of function, and divided into orthodox 'systems'. These are really classes of tissue whose components are histologically or functionally similar. Neurologists, for example, are therefore firstly experts in properties of nervous tissue. In cases of gross pathological disturbance and/or the need for surgery, the positional relationships become more important in proportion as abnormal interference ensues between structures of different 'systems' (for example, erosion of or pressure on structures by neoplasms). It is as if the subtleties of regional anatomy are lost to the charms of basic physiology.

The orthodox 'systemic' divisions are reflected in the various hospital departmental divisions (cardiology, endocrinology, gastroenterology, neurology, urology, orthopaedics, etc). These divisions are now necessary more in order to house the peculiar requirements of extreme expertise, rather than to emphasise the historic, attitudinal compartmentalisation of the body.

Manual therapy, rather than beginning body-analysis in terms of function, instead may begin with a reduction into regions of the body, such as the head and neck. These regions are seen as organised zones — true systems. The components of such a system, therefore, as previously stated, together with their physiological properties, acquire an anatomical positional context first and foremost. Naturally, the functionally similar features of orthodox 'systems' or classes are considered by manual practitioners. But this is only after a consideration of their value in the positional system. The reason for this is that *physiological features are considered to be capable of alteration and modification by the effects of the positional relationships in the true system.* Consequently, systemic position is the ground context in which physiological functioning is to be considered. The emphasis of treatment is therefore on zones that are related by virtue of physiologically significant arrangement.

This conceptual distinction reflects an attitudinal contrast between, especially, osteopathic manual therapists and orthodoxy. The systems view is held to be a more accurate and useful model of how the body is organised than one based firstly upon distinct physiological characteristics.

Further examples

1. Ordinarily, the proximity of the twelfth rib and its associated myofascial structures on the one hand (a subsystem), and the kidney on the other (a subsystem), is significant in terms only of geographical knowledge. This becomes important in the case of gross pathological disturbance of one system by the other, and especially by the need for surgery. For manual practitioners, however, significance is to be found in those mechanical and physiological relationships existing between these two subsystems, and between them and their immediate suprasystem (the system of the abdomen). This latter kind of understanding is considered to be of importance fundamentally in conceptualising about the human organism, and not simply in cases of gross pathology.

2. The relationship between the sternocleidomastoid muscles and the mid-cervical facet joint cartilages is considered significant. It is mechanically significant because hypertonia of the former will impose new mechanical conditions upon the latter. It is physiologically significant because these new conditions, if unremitting, may facilitate adaptive, or even degenerative changes in the cartilage, periosteum, and related structures.

3. The system of the head and neck and the system of the thorax can be considered subsystems of a greater whole system. Long-term restriction and depression of the upper, anterior portion of the ribcage, protraction of the glenohumeral and scapulothoracic joints and increased thoracic kyphosis and cervical lordosis will impose mechanical limitation on the range of movement on cervical fascial connective tissue. This influence would extend to all cervical epineural and epivascular connective tissue. Since these latter tissues are contin-

uous with both intra- and extracranial dura, periosteum and certain cranial nerve epineuria, then the stressful mechanical forces initiated in the thorax will be transmitted to these structures. The fact that this might be a reasonable description of a series of mechanical relationships is a fact of the true systemic view. It merely describes some of the anatomical continuities between the chest and the base of the brain, and concludes that mechanical stresses in the former will be transmitted to the latter. This in itself is not a staggering revelation. It depends for its significance upon the validity of premise one. That is, it depends upon the extent to which physiological functioning of the latter tissues will be compromised by the new mechanical conditions. These kinds of force transmission are, by and large, simply excluded from orthodox medical theory. Their physiological influence is in need of investigation. If the systems view is valid, it would require a review of the science of pathophysiology.

Currently, both in medical schools and schools of manual medicine, the teaching of anatomy is often divided into regional anatomy (that of the forearm, the hand, etc), and systemic anatomy (that of 'systems'; myology, neurology, arthrology, osteology, etc). A more useful nomenclature based upon this analysis would therefore be *systemic anatomy* for the former kind, and *anatomy by tissue class* for the latter.

Psychological implications of systems theory

The above account has emphasised organisation between systems. But systems theory rests also upon the notion of hierarchical organisation, commonly depicted using concentric circles (Fig. 2.1). Just as the understanding of a knee joint is considerably enhanced by placing it within the context of the entire lower extremity, and just as the understanding of a child's behaviour is considerably enhanced by placing him in the context of familial relationships, so the understanding of any system within the body is enhanced by placing it within a larger context. For example, the context of the patient's intended activity is a fitting context in which to place the study of any particular physiological event. The quality of action is subject to physical and physiological idiosyncrasies peculiar to the patient's character. For example, the quality and degree of persistence of arousal

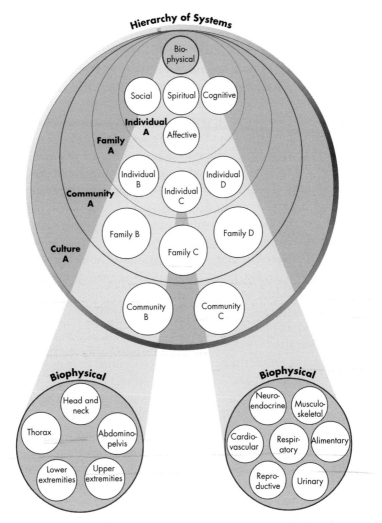

Figure 2.1 Hierarchical organisation of systems, showing examples of further subsystems within the biophysical domain. (Adapted from Schuster & Ashburn 1980. Reprinted by permission of Lippincott Williams and Wilkins.)

(sympathetico-adrenomedullary and pituitary-adrenocortical) is character dependent. Patients' emotional states and volitional dispositions will determine the exact nature of any activity, just as much as beliefs and concepts will. Since these qualities are unique to each individual, then a fuller understanding of a physiological event will arise from viewing it in the context of such qualities.

This is clearly a complicated task. So-called 'holistic' or contextual attitudes towards healing are inevitably more elaborate and involved than their more reductionistic counterparts. Nevertheless, an appreciation of systems theory demands a consideration of those aspects of the suprasystems that appear relevant to the case. Appropriate suprasystems can be chosen from long-term or short-term constitutional and circumstantial phenomena. For example, a particular bodily disorder can be placed within a context of features of emotional character, sex, cultural world view, etc. These can be further 'contained' within the suprasystems of sexual and other relationships, family role, home, workplace and so on. The essential point here is that such contexts are considered relevant directly as a result of the use of systems theory in the understanding of the organisation of human beings.

The physicist David Bohm (1917–1992) argued that the habit of analysis by dividing into constituent parts is only one method of analysing structures or functions. Instead of splitting wholes up into parts and studying parts (which results, naturally enough, in the study of parts rather than wholes), wholes can be analysed in terms of *what they are a part of.* Similarly, a tree cannot be defined only as a structure with roots at one end and leaves at the other, because the molecular interchange between air and leaves at one end, and earth and roots at the other is evidence of the tree's interdependence with a greater suprasystem. It is the failure to recognise the interdependence of systems and suprasystems that can lead, in this case, to environmental destruction. Similarly, account of a person's bodily parts without placing them into their physical, psychological and environmental suprasystems may be followed by a lack of respect for the person.

More specific attributes of systems such as human beings or the subsystems within them have been suggested by Schuster & Ashburn (1980):

1. The components of the system and the resultant boundaries.
2. The suprasystem, environment, resources and constraints of the system.
3. The relationship between the components and the efficiency of the communication system.

Knowing the abdomin – requires many physiological levels and subsystems + emotional, personal, attitudinal, cultural, historical awareness

IS MANUAL THERAPY ONLY TECHNOLOGY AND PROCEDURE?   **59**

4. The *objectives* or *goals* of the total system.
5. The *roles* or *responsibilities* of the *component subsystems* and the *efficiency with which the subsystems carry out their responsibilities*.
6. The *management component* of the system.
7. The *history* or *time-perspective of the system*.'
   (Schuster & Ashburn 1980 pp 35–36)

A consideration of these attributes again requires attention to neurological, psychological and ultimately larger environmental contexts. This is necessary when considering attributes 4, 5, 6 and 7 and not merely 2.

The *systems view*, then, since it insists that things can only be known fully when in the context of the highest relevant suprasystem, *requires* a knowledge of psychological and emotional concepts in order to understand bodily subsystems fully. A system of forearm muscles, for example, in addition to other physiological properties, requires an understanding of the peripheral and central nervous system. The latter is, likewise, placed in the context of the suprasystem of character, which, in turn, resides in and has been formed in, various relationships — interpersonal and otherwise.

Systems theory implicates the relevance of wholes. If it, as a model, fits manual therapy theory, then manual therapy too implicates wholes — the psychological-in-context, and not merely the mechanical.
¿ spiritual & mental (eg unconscious mind)

THE INTEREST IN MUSCLES

If the manual practitioner's concept of muscle function is essentially contextual, then the usual account of muscle function merely in terms of property is deficient. For example, the function of the biceps muscle, rather than to contract, is to:

- flex the elbow joint
- supinate the elbow joint
- help stabilise the shoulder joint
- raise a stiff sash window
- put up 20 shelves in one day
- lift a beer glass every evening
- shake a fist (express an emotion)

- attract (some) women
- win weight-lifting competitions.

Good functioning of a muscle, as far as the patient is concerned, will depend upon what she, idiosyncratically, requires of it. The practitioner's attention to it must always bear in mind this particular need. This contextual functioning is distinct from properties of muscle tissue, which could be described largely in terms of physiology.

Understanding muscle function merely as elaborate self-righting biochemical machinery, explainable in terms of mechanistic preceding causes, is a contracted view. This is firstly because such functions are really properties of people and not inanimate chemical systems, as described above. But in the case of muscle functioning, which contributes more to self-expression and self-assertion than to mere self-persistence (see premise two), the appropriateness of a teleological, contextual view becomes much more obvious.

Manual practitioners place special importance upon the muscular and skeletal tissues of the body. There are sound physiological reasons for this unorthodox shift in attitude. For example, the musculo-skeletal tissues are the users of the most blood and energy in the body. Furthermore, the utilisation of these resources is enormously variable. This indicates that the muscular tissues considered as a whole comprise a hugely adaptable homeostatic reservoir. Muscles therefore produce significant effects upon the total body economy and other subsystems. The significance of having to lie down when ill, for example, is that muscular tissues utilise vast energy resources whilst upright. During illness they must relinquish their thirst for these resources. Energy can then be used by self-regulation and self-defence processes recruited for healing.

Movement is personal

There is also deep symbolic significance in the musculoskeletal tissues. People express their humanity with their movement. Irvin Korr, a prominent physiologist, points out that life does not consist of ventricular contraction, glomerular filtration and Krebs cycle. It consists of walking, talking, sitting, eating, working, loving and fighting, that is, expression through muscular movement. Each person demonstrates who she is and what she feels and believes in, by how she holds herself, stands, moves, writes, speaks. Personality, intellect, imagination, creativity, perceptions, love, compassion, values and philosophies are finally manifested through muscular movement (Korr 1970, 1997).

Movement expresses life. The muscular tissues are the moving tissues. They move according to how our lives are lived and deserve special attention as agents of our essence. The muscular tissues are the tools of the soul, as it were. Wittgenstein wrote 'the human body is the best picture of the human soul' (Wittgenstein 1974). The muscular and skeletal components of the body are the most massive, most outwardly obvious, most immediately recognisable ones.

Because bodily movement expresses human life more intelligibly than biochemistry, then manual practitioners are keen to use theories of motion as a contextual framework for their work. A recognition of this notion in the minds of patients may go some way to explain the recent growth of the manual therapy professions. One person's movement characteristics are suggestive of her*self*, her personal identity, and not merely of biochemistry. This symbolic and phenomenological view of the kinetic qualities of body systems is outside the principles of premise one, but is explored in later chapters. It is included here to shed more light on why manual practitioners are especially interested in the muscular and skeletal tissues, and not only from the point of view of their role as muscular tissue specialists. This well-known aspect of osteopathic theory is an example of an area in which it consciously moves out of the realms of physiology. It demonstrates once again the immediate link between muscle physiology and the emotive life of which it partakes.

A person's 'humanity' is, by and large, not considered to be represented by a collection of mechanical phenomena. Rather, it is considered in terms of teleological and value-laden ideas such as moral and emotive thought. But if manual practitioners are dealing directly with those tissues by which a person lives out her 'humanity', then it seems sensible to explore how such themes should be accounted for in theories of manual health care.

Another psychologically relevant aspect of 'musclology' (which is the 'study of muscles') is the development of palpable muscle hypertonia by the unconscious mind. Words such as 'uptight', 'tense' and 'jumpy' are in fact physical descriptions arising from the effect of anxiety on the neuromuscular system. As such they have become incorporated into colloquial usage as metaphors for anxiety. Emotionally generated muscle hypertonia is dramatic evidence of a psychological context for muscle function. This is discussed further in Chapter 4.

THE IMPORTANCE OF THE INTERVERTEBRAL SEGMENT TO MANIPULATIVE THERAPY

One of the fundamental claims of both chiropractic and osteopathic theory is that there is a spinal segmental component to disease processes. In fact the greater part of the theoretical contribution from these disciplines, especially from chiropractic, is in terms of spinal segmental dysfunction. (These theories will not be analysed in detail here, and the reader is referred to standard texts, eg Haldeman 1992, Ward 1997).

Early chiropractic texts are very clear on the point that the essence of the chiropractic approach is to correct subluxations of vertebral and other bony tissues, thereby creating proper alignment and balance in the bony structures. A subluxation was considered to be a vertebral segment that is not frankly dislocated, but is out of normal anatomic relationship to the adjacent segments. Decrease in motion was and is considered to be one of the key features of subluxations, which are thought to involve nerve transmission changes largely through pressure effects. Such changes impair normal functioning, contributing significantly towards pathogenic change in tissue supplied by affected nerves. The mediating factor between the subluxation and the disease is therefore thought to be the nervous system. A structural problem, usually within the spine or pelvis, can, it is thought, contribute to diminished neurologic ability to cope with the environment. The ability of the body to heal itself is consequently decreased (Haldeman 1992, p 32).

Since these ideas were first articulated, there has been much debate concerning the nature and origin of the subluxation, and a wealth of theoretic speculation concerning both its significance and the effects of manipulation upon it. The general consensus is, however, that the chiropractor aims to correct what the body seems unable to, so that the innate intelligence, or inherent healing force, is able once again to operate unimpeded.

With respect to vertebral segmental disorder, it is fair to say that osteopathic theory would largely concur with these ideas — perhaps with emphasis upon functional rather than structural disorder. Chiropractic texts emphasise peripheral nerve compression effects of abnormal structural relationships. Osteopathic texts tend to emphasise functional changes and inter/motorneurone hyperexcitability or facilitation (long-term sensitisation). Whereas the founder of chiropractic, D D Palmer, emphasised nerve function as being that which is essentially disturbed by subluxation, the founder of osteopathy, A T Still, often emphasised vascular effects of mechanical disorder. Since nerves receive vasa nervorum, and blood vessels sympathetic nervi vasorum, it may be necessary to recognise the cyclical nature of these claims.

The osteopathic segmental lesion, although described in terms that differ from the chiropractic one, should nevertheless be considered identically in terms of physiology. Regardless of whether or not bony misalignments, aberrant mobility characteristics, nociception or whatever are responsible for spinal segmental dysfunction, both professions pay much attention to the correction of it (although osteopaths probably concern themselves less with it than with the concept of bodily structural faults in general). But it is not useful to make clear distinctions between the professions with respect to theoretical minutiae of these kinds (even if texts suggest them), since intra- and inter-professional practice is highly variable.

Both chiropractic and osteopathic texts often make the important point that practitioners need not concern themselves with particular disease processes, or ailments, especially as described by orthodox classifications. This is because the manipulative procedures are methods of treatment applicable to any patient. It is thought necessary merely to locate relevant structural/functional disturbances and endeavour to correct them. In doing so, practitioners are attempting to influence positively those aberrant neurological, vascular and vital mechanisms contributing to disease processes.

Spinal reflexes

The degree of sensitivity of muscular tissue to the neurological information it receives is variable, and is determined by both central and peripheral nervous systems. The organisation of this sensitivity is achieved partly by means of a series of reflexes operating in a cyclic continuum from central nervous system to periphery and back again. But 'horizontally organised' systems such as these reflexes are ultimately controlled by stimulatory and inhibitory influences from 'longitudinal', centrally ordered and highly patterned, unconscious neurological mechanisms.

Both healthy and unhealthy reflex systems rely in part upon cues from receptor stations in the muscles, joint capsules, fascias and in other soft tissues. The receptors report according to the velocity and de/acceleration of stretch of, and pressure in, those tissues — that is, upon mechanical factors. It has been proposed that persistent noxious stimuli (biochemical or mechanical) can alter the neurological 'volume control' of muscular irritability at a central level. The threshold of interneurone and motorneurone excitability appears to become lowered and the area is said to be facilitated. The condition gives rise to functional disorders characterised by inappropriate properties of mobility, tone and often discomfort.

Osteopaths have argued that certain manual techniques could be used to treat these functional disorders by decreasing abnormal neurological irritability at the spinal level. This is said to be achieved by virtue of the specific effects of different rates and intensities of passive movements (in the spine and periphery) upon interneurone and motorneurone irritability — ie treating the reflex system. Whilst it is likely that manual treatment can influence local peripheral tissue factors giving rise to altered proprioception and nociception, the notion that manual treatment can influence neurological motor tone has recently been seriously challenged (Lederman 1997, ch. 8).

Spinal segmental facilitation was first proposed as a mechanism capable of contributing to the development of both visceral and nonvisceral disorder in the first part of the 20th century. Osteopaths have usually assumed that their success in treating such disorders was based upon normalising these aberrant reflex patterns through the local effects of manipulation. The basis of this assumption is that long-term sensitisation of segmental reflex systems is considered to be independent of higher influences (Patterson & Wurster 1997). But Lederman (1997) has argued that the normalisation of these disorders by the stimulation of reflex systems cannot take place because the higher, central motor system determinants would not be sufficiently addressed. Lederman contends that long-term motor dysfunction is a neurologically learned phenomenon and cannot resolve without active (volitional) and cognitive processes. Lederman uses the term 'guidance' to describe how manual treatment can aid these rehabilitation processes. He insists that purely passive techniques, with the patient in a completely relaxed state, cannot influence the motor system.

It is important to realise that a very large proportion of osteopaths have nevertheless relied upon the concept of segmental reflex treatment in their practices. This has been for the treatment of both visceral disorder by virtue of viscero-somatic and somato-visceral reflexes, and for the treatment of non-visceral disorder. Lederman is not challenging the existence of facilitation of spinal reflexes, but the notion that manual techniques can be used to treat them using reflex stimulation. Such a challenge targets one of the central tenets of modern osteopathy.

Lederman goes on to stress that, if patients' nervous systems cannot be controlled by peripheral events, then techniques should be used that involve the patient actively and cognitively shaping a motor learning response with the guidance of the practitioner (Lederman 1997, chs. 9, 10). This is a far cry from the typical image of the passive patient, in relative ignorance, being manipulated.

The majority of osteopaths and chiropractors do not, however, utilise active and cognitive techniques as the mainstay of their treatments. Therefore, if Lederman's crushing blow to reflex theory is correct, there must be other explanations for the obvious efficacy of treatment. If the effect of manipulation upon dysfunctional motorneurone pools is not mediated peripherally, it must be mediated by higher centres. That is, the effects of manipulation upon peripheral and spinal neural systems are likely to be brought about by psychological events.

Lederman concedes this by, as mentioned above, insisting upon the necessity of the patient's active and cognitive involvement in manual processes. But it is more significant that he devotes a third of his entire text to 'Psychological and psychophysiological processes in manual therapy'. In this chapter he discusses the value of largely unconscious psychological events influencing the outcome of manual therapy. Lederman's work, therefore, is heavily supportive of the thesis of this book, despite his initial detailed analysis of physiological mechanisms.

It should be pointed out here that non-neurological rationales explaining manual therapy are not affected by Lederman's criticisms. Those effects of manipulation upon peripheral tissue brought about by facilitating, repair processes, improvement in mechanical features of tissues and improvement in blood, lymph and synovial fluid dynamics will likely decrease afferent neurological noise and contribute to a feeling of well-being. But where manipulative theory is centred around spinal segmental neurology, as much of modern osteopathic and chiropractic theory is, then it must proceed with caution; much research is needed.

Manual therapy and psychiatry, and the psychological implications of segmentology

Chiropractic

Despite the reliance upon mechanical concepts, psychological components of disease are mentioned at the outset in both chiropractic and osteopathic texts. The early chiropractors firmly believed that manipulation could cure mental problems because the treatment removed neurological and vascular impediments to the expression of the life force. This innate intelligence, when permitted to operate unimpeded, allowed the individual to better himself physically, mentally and spiritually (Haldeman 1992, p 32). 'It is only necessary to let the innate express itself and everything the person does will be functionally ideal' (Waagen & Strang 1992). In reality, despite the fact that psychological factors were believed capable of contributing to dysfunction (see, eg; Haldeman 1992, p 37, on the work of W D Harper), the treatment of choice was nevertheless manipulation. Willard Carver, one of the foremost chiropractic theoreticians, believed that suggestion was the basis of all systems of medicine, since the same percentage of cures was to be found throughout all of them. He believed treatment should be aimed at removing those structural impediments that prevented the effects of suggestion from influencing, via the nervous system, the entire body (Haldeman 1992, p 38). Modern chiropractic admits to the holistic, vitalistic and untestable principle of the innate, although it emphasises the scientific for explanations.

Schwartz's *Mental Health and Chiropractic — a Multidisciplinary Approach* (1973) sets out the place for chiropractic treatment in psychiatry, beginning: 'For the first time, chiropractic is fully explored as a possible treatment for emotional distress when such distress is due to spinal subluxations. The possible stressful reactions that stem from spinal subluxations and the physiological and psychological improvements that can occur from their correction, have far-reaching and significant effects upon the total organism.' Directly psychological effects are mentioned, especially those brought about by the relationship between practitioner and patient. The psychologically satisfying and confidence-building effects upon the patient of the physical, active and direct nature of manipulative strategies are discussed in brief. But the thrust of the entire text centres on the detrimental effects of spinal subluxations upon the psyche, and the benefits of removing such defects.

Osteopathy

A T Still, the founder of osteopathy, gave this formal definition of his creation:

> 'Osteopathy is that science which consists of such exact, exhaustive and verifiable knowledge of the structure and function of the human mechanism, anatomical, physiological and psychological, including the chemistry and physics of its known elements, as has made discoverable certain organic laws and remedial resources, within the body itself, by which nature under the scientific treatment peculiar to osteopathic practice, apart from ordinary methods of extraneous artificial or medicinal stimulation, and in harmonious accord with its own mechanical principles, molecular activities, and metabolic processes, may recover from displacements, disorganisations, derangements, and consequent disease, and regain its normal equilibrium of form and function in health and strength.' (Still 1908, p 403)

This highly enigmatic ('certain organic laws') but essentially mechanico-physical account refers to the psychological in terms of its structure and function. It allows for the mechanical correction of displacements, disorganisations and derangements, thereby assisting 'nature's' (ie the innate's) recovery of health. The psychological is in there, but couched in mechanistic terms. Still himself sometimes directed his physical work specifically at the patient's psyche (Still 1908, p 112).

Only 20 years after the founding of the first school of osteopathy in Kirksville, Missouri, the Still–Hildreth Osteopathic Sanatorium was established in Macon in the same state. This is clear testimony to the perceived efficacy of osteopathic manipulation in the area of psychiatry. Floyd Dunn published, in 1948, The Osteopathic Management of Psychosomatic Problems. In this paper, Dunn carefully and insightfully states not merely the effects of treatment upon visceral disorders such as gastric ulcer and cardiac dysrhythmia, which were considered to be produced by the combination of anxiety and somatic factors, but also the directly psychological effects, worth quoting here in full:

> '1. *The reassurance of manual contact. In the minds of all of us are old memories, placed there in earliest childhood, of the comfort and security which was ours when our mothers' warm and loving hands soothed away our childish troubles or fears. Remember that in periods of illness, we tend to retrogress emotionally toward the relatively simpler and more secure time of our childhood, and that when the illness is largely emotional in nature this retrogression is proportionately more pronounced. The patient is therefore prepared by his illness to receive favourably and to benefit psychologically by the ministrations of his osteopathic physician.*
>
> 2. *The effect of physical operation. The fact that the osteopathic physician "does something" to the patient's body has its psychological effect entirely apart from the more purely physiological responses which result from such manual operations. Each of us has a mental concept of his physical body, which in psychiatric parlance is termed "the body image". As the physician proceeds with his manipulations, the patient sees and feels his body structure being altered and makes corresponding favourable changes in his mental image of himself.*

3. *The mental effect of diminished skeletal muscular tension. This effect
   needs no elaboration. We are all familiar with the diminution of
   emotional tension consequent upon the muscular relaxation which
   always follows proper osteopathic manipulative therapy.*
4. *The mental effect of improved visceral function. The sense of well-
   being accompanying proper visceral function is likewise too familiar
   to the osteopathic physician to need explanation. Nor do I think it
   necessary to elaborate upon the point that osteopathic therapy will
   improve visceral function if correctly applied.*
5. *The effect of care and attention. It is always a source of ego-satisfaction
   to be the recipient of the care and attention of someone for whom we
   have a feeling of respect and high regard. The very fact that giving
   osteopathic manipulative treatments takes time and effort on the part
   of the physician is gratifying to the patient's sense of personal
   importance, and thus is bound to have a beneficial psychological
   effect.'* (Dunn 1948)

Other articles on the subject of manual treatment in psychiatry have
emerged, for example Dunn (1950, 1952) and Bradford (1965). Bradford,
although admitting and adding to those ideas proposed initially by
Dunn, takes pains to explain, along a similar vein to the early chiropractic texts, how peripheral afferents can contribute to central nervous
system disorder and hence emotional disorder. Gellhorn (1964) concurs
with this view, although noting the paradoxical finding that 'increased
proprioceptive discharges induced by passive movements increase sympathetic discharges and, via the hypothalamus, the state of alertness'.
One wonders exactly what manner of passive movements were admin-
istered during this research in the light of Bradford's comment that
'rhythmic stimulation of the ordinary sensory receptors has been utilised
as a calming measure since the dawn of history' (Bradford 1965, p 485).

Bradford, however, completes an overview of the *directly* psychological effects of manipulation in under three columns. He concludes:
'if the advantages of osteopathic treatment for these [emotional] disorders lay solely in the realm of the psychologic, its benefits, though
considerable, would be decidedly limited'. He then presses on with
the local physiological effects of manipulation pertinent to reducing
cerebral irritation for the following 13 columns.

R Hope Robertson (*c* 1938) when talking about his success with schizophrenic patients, dogmatically states: '[the] fundamental principle of osteopathic treatment is the correcting of physical causes, which, through their adverse influence on the autonomic nervous system, bring about disturbed [cerebral] circulation, the underlying factor of this disease'. Hope Robertson claimed he could cure at least 62% of thoroughly representative cases of 2 years' standing, and 90% of cases taken in their early stages.

In the main, treatment techniques were considered to cause physiological relaxation of skeletal muscle, which reduces bodily tension, and relaxes the patient. Treatment was also considered to reduce spinal irritation of both somatic and visceral autonomic systems. This would thereby contribute to the resolution of physical symptoms predisposed by spinal segmental facilitation and precipitated by anxiety. The quietening of nociception and the decrease in other inappropriate peripheral afferents achieved with manipulation were considered to cause a decrease in the overall afferent neurological noise, previously contributing to irritation at a psychological level (see items 3 and 4 in Dunn 1948, quoted above). In summary, treatment was considered both to ease the neurological load on higher centres from the periphery, and to ease the anxiety-induced peripheral irritation *by* higher centres. It was also considered to be capable of improving cerebral circulation.

Where the effects of manipulation were speculated upon in any detail by these authors, they were couched very largely in terms of spinal segmental reflex neurology. Again, if Lederman's criticisms of those explanations cited above are correct, then it is necessary to conclude that treatment has primarily a deeply psychologically relaxing effect, and a centrally ordered effect upon spinal motor learning events. These are then translated into a global reduction in muscular tone, and decrease in interneurone and motorneurone pool irritability. Lederman states that 'controlling the motor systems via the activation of peripheral mechanisms and segmental reflexes is equivalent to attempting to change the flow of a river by throwing a pebble into it'. Such a metaphor appears even more appropriate when considering the treatment of psychological problems with manual therapy. Dunn's directly psychological effects may be more extensive and important in the treatment of both psychological and physical disorder than has previously been thought.

Physiotherapy

It should be noted that, despite its inclusion in orthodoxy, physiotherapy has by no means always been used in psychiatric and psychosomatic medicine. Nevertheless, advanced physical therapy modes specifically addressing the problems of anxiety and stress, psychosomasis, and psychiatric disturbances in general have emerged. These include psychomotor therapy, body awareness therapy, integrated respiration therapy, and the use of autogenic training in physiotherapeutic settings. These particular disciplines are described in *Psychological and Psychosomatic Problems* (Hegna & Sveram 1990), which includes a chapter on the integration of psychological factors in the physical treatment of post-traumatic stress.

These disciplines are practised by a small minority of the profession. They emphasise the indivisibility of mind and body, the relevance of emotions to the development of bodily disorders and recovery from them, the central importance of the patient/practitioner relationship, and the need for self-development and maturity in the practitioner. As a generic group — albeit with greatly differing therapeutic styles — these and associated disciplines encourage in the patient: responsibility, self-confidence, self-awareness and relaxation skills. Because it is acknowledged that an individual is always both mind and body simultaneously, patients are helped to understand and explore how their own feelings and attitudes have influenced their body language, self-image, posture, movement patterns and symptom development.

Another comprehensive — if more orthodox — text is *Physiotherapy in Mental Health* (Everett et al 1995). This includes chapters on physiological aspects of stress, stress management, relaxation training, exercise and movement therapy and, significantly, a useful chapter on touch, handling and non-verbal communication. The book is largely concerned with practical aspects of physiotherapy in a variety of settings ranging from child psychiatry through eating disorders and substance abuse, to post-traumatic stress and dementia. Unlike its less orthodox colleagues osteopathy and chiropractic (with few exceptions), it is fair to say that such physiotherapy theory is, in general, broader, and more humanistic in its approach to the considerations of psychological issues in physical therapy. This may well be partly because the educative role in physiotherapy is well established, perhaps in proportion as the amount of direct manual involvement has decreased. This allows physiotherapists to avoid placing patients in too passive a role, and promotes their cognitive involvement and self-reliance. However, in common with its manipulative colleagues, physiotherapy has paid scant attention to researching the psychological significance of manual contact.

MASSAGE AND NON-NEUROLOGICAL PHYSIOLOGICAL EFFECTS OF MANUAL THERAPY

The physiotherapy profession started life as The Society of Trained Masseuses, established in 1894 by a group of nurses and midwives practising 'medical rubbing' (Poon 1995). They, in common with massage therapists in general, might lay claim to a therapeutic modality sporting a pedigree considerably more ancient than manipulation. The profession as a whole has tended to move away from purely manual work in the direction of exercise prescription and the embracing of the technological specialisation inherent in modern physical therapy. However, the founders expected that the profession would always be associated with manual expertise (Williams 1986).

The physiological effects of massage therapy and other rhythmic bodywork, including joint mobilisation, can be described in terms of:

- techniques which enhance tissue repair
- techniques which alter the mechanical behaviour of tissue
- techniques which improve fluid movement (Lederman 1997, p. 55).

Such theories serve to augment the neurological and mechanical principles outlined elsewhere in this chapter. Improving comfort in tissue by such techniques will undoubtedly improve the patient's sense of well-being, by decreasing the degree to which the self is irritated by noxious somatic sensations. However, the degree to which manual techniques directly improve the patient's sense of well-being and thereby promote the resolution of peripheral problems has tended to be put aside.

There is much evidence that touch and massage-type techniques are capable of producing beneficial physiological effects, within the body, both generally, and in specific instances of disorder. Massage therapists of all varieties have always noted the relaxing effects, above all others, of this form of treatment, and the overall feeling of well-being that good massage always brings about. It is perhaps in massage more than in any other form of manual treatment that is to be found the suspicion that psychological effects are probably more at play than purely local physiological ones.

Massage therapists always promote their work by drawing attention to the ability of massage to relieve stress and tension by inducing physiological relaxation. Research into the effects of the relaxation response upon nociception, sympathetic arousal, immune competence and healing in general is likely to reinforce the notion that central, psychologically mediated events help to resolve peripheral disorders, rather than the other way around.

Gjertrud Roxendal's thoughts (Roxendal 1990) on certain psychological aspects of massage serve to consolidate some of these ideas:

'1. *Massage is communication. The therapist takes care and sends messages, especially the question: "How are you?" The patient receives the care and answers by reactions in breathing, muscular tension and reactions in the skin.*

2. *Massage confirms the person (the receiver) through his body. The fact that the therapist agrees to touch the patient includes an aspect of accepting him as a person.*

3. *Massage can stimulate inner processes. A rhythmic pressure directed towards deep levels of the body can stimulate processes such as postural activity, breathing and digestion.*

4. *Massage can reduce both muscular and inner tension. It is not necessary to give relaxing massage as local therapy. Tension headache is often reduced by foot massage or treatment on the calf muscles.*

5. *Massage can lead to passivity and regression of the patient. Relaxation and rest can increase the patient's access to his resources, but it might also make the patient passive and dependent. In these cases massage should temporarily be avoided, or maybe combined with independent exercise.*

6. *Massage can stimulate the body's production of endorphins. This increases the feeling of well-being and is pain-relieving.*
7. *Massage can lead to increased tension in hypotonic muscles. Techniques for this purpose are being developed in, for example, Norway.*
8. *There are techniques which work with special tissues or are directed towards autonomic reflexes. Correctly used, however, they influence the whole body and the patient's psychic life.'* (Roxendal 1990, p 94)

This has not been a review of the literature concerning the physiological effects of manual therapy, but rather a brief exploration of what questions may be begged if such a review were to be undertaken in detail. Does the available literature present a balanced view of what manual therapy actually achieves, or can achieve? Important psychological issues emerge from a consideration of most if not all manual therapy theories. This suggests that the available literature is unsuitably biased in favour of physiological explanations and the body-as-machine view.

Grieve's *Modern Manual Therapy* (Boyling & Palastanga 1994), probably the most highly respected text on manual therapy, considers the failure by modern medicine to treat successfully and halt the rising cost and disruption to lifestyle wrought by benign spinal pain syndromes. It admits that 'no single treatment seems to be more successful than any other — or more successful than natural history and the placebo effect' (Zusman 1994). This admission is placed at the conclusion of a chapter which begins: 'Important elements intrinsic to the patient–practitioner encounter, such as reassurance, expectations, confidence, enthusiasm, beliefs, perceptions and the so-called placebo effect are not considered here'. The tendency of mainstream literature to ignore so-called unscientific subjects, even though they have been shown to be at least as important as the factors normally included, is regrettable.

MANIPULATION AS PROCEDURAL TOUCHING

Touch is used by manual practitioners in order to gather part of the information necessary for making a diagnostic judgement. It is also used for treatment. What kind of touching is this?

The kind of touching implied by the mechanico-physical theories described above is 'procedural' or 'instrumental' touch. The familiar analogy is between the body and a complex machine and the therapy is therefore analogous to engineering. Typically, during treatment, a series of procedures will be used such as: soft-tissue kneading, rhythmic articulation, thrusting movements, traction, multidimensional compression, and so on. These procedures are carried out on an object — body tissue — as if it were a machine. Indeed manual therapy relies on the fact that body tissue does have certain features in common with a machine. For example, one can identify levers, bevels, pivots, hinges and ball-and-sockets.

The attitude to body tissue in manual therapy is the same as that in surgery — although clearly manual therapy is less invasive, less painful, and performed on a conscious patient. The perspective is the same: flesh cannot sufficiently be influenced by the patient's psyche to render manipulation (surgery) unnecessary. Furthermore, flesh is actual, physical stuff which can be acted upon — unlike the intangible self. Its physical characteristics are thereby alterable by such action.

In common with other medical practices such as incisions, ultrasound investigations, steroid injections, femoral stabs and reflex testing, manual practitioners appear to be performing techniques upon flesh — lateral fluctuations, high-velocity thrusts, adjustments, muscle-energy, counter-strains and harmonic technique. This kind of touching is characteristic of modern health care and is utterly distinct from the common, everyday use of touching as a form of self-expression and self-assertion. That is, it is distinct from the kind of touch that takes place during non-verbal communication. A notable exception in a modern health care setting is when a nurse holds a patient's hand during a painful medical procedure, and other similar examples.

The Cartesian ground for scientific medical thought allows for manipulation to be considered as wholly procedural. This is because the body is typically seen as both separate from and different to the mind or soul. Indeed, body tissue is considered sufficiently divorced from the person to enable procedures to be carried out on a patient's flesh with the patient looking on, as it were. This renders the patient a passive innocent bystander somehow divorced from, but nevertheless chained to, the terrain of the therapeutic battle. If the patient could leave the clinic and return to collect her body when the treatment is finished, she probably would elect to do so. Patients, too, therefore, hold the belief that their bodies are machines, prone to the occasional incomprehensible breakdown, and at such times in need of fixing. It is inconvenient for patients to be present whilst the engineers carry out their service, but they have no choice.

'Doing things to', rather than 'doing things with' or 'being with' patients, emphasises the mechanical at the expense of the personal. Procedural touch invokes the inanimate as the object of its actions. This is in part because the passivity inherent in being acted upon is more a characteristic of the inanimate than of the animate. But it is also because techniques are associated with technology, whose objects are by and large non-human.

It is noteworthy that where physiological theories for manual health care approaches are absent, such as in the 'laying on of hands' for example, the type of touching cannot be described as being purely technical or procedural. Instead, there is a sense of communication implied in the act, or some notion of the touching as facilitating a more direct contact — 'in touch' with the patient-as-person. In fact there is an underlying assumption that, if the type of touching is a *technique*, then there would not be the 'whole person' effect implicit, for example, in the 'laying on of hands'.

Practitioners, of course, do not treat their *patients* as if they were inanimate machines, but they do treat their *bodies* as if they were. There is no doubt that this attitude to treatment and bodies has its rightful place. The majority of practitioners show respect, care and empathy to the person, whilst at the same time treating a body. But treating bodies is what they do, because they are not (at least as far as they are aware) psychotherapists.

TREATING PEOPLE — NOT BODIES?

If manual practitioners merely treat people's bodies (and bodily disorders are just that — only bodily) then the current physiological rationales suffice, at least for the time being. But despite the foregoing demonstration that manual practitioners treat people's bodies, nevertheless they frequently claim to treat 'the whole person' (in common with other perpetrators of the holistic approach). If this is the case, they ought to be able to describe their work in the context of a philosophical framework showing that people are essentially their bodies rather than essentially their minds or personalities. In which case treating the body would be treating the person.

However, it is important to realise that a wholly materialistic framework, such as the one currently assumed by orthodox medicine, is unsuitable for this purpose, despite the fact that it proposes that mental phenomena are reducible to physico-chemical events. It is unsuitable because the concept of a person-as-body is impossible to explain in mechanico-physiological terms. This is because attributes of a person make much better sense if they are explained in quite different terms (see Ch. 1). The way in which a person *is* his body, and therefore the way in which bodily treatment is treatment of the person, is not, using the mechanical paradigm, possible to describe. This is why the innate intelligence idea is so useful in manual medicine, since it includes the person and his inherent ability to function and expresses himself (so long as his structure is integrated). The presence of the innate frees the manipulator to concentrate on the physical, allowing the mental and emotional to be taken care of by the improved flow of the 'life force'.

Manual therapy as whole-person therapy perhaps needs to show how people's physical, tactile lives form the ground of their experience as human beings. This would necessitate a phenomenological description of the effect of manual therapy on the psyche-in-the-body, or on the 'lived body'. Phenomenology is suitable because it refuses to consider the body in the same way as other material stuff, as Descartes (1972) insisted it is: 'the fire which burns continually in the heart ... is of no other nature than all those fires that occur in inanimate bodies'. Phenomenology points out that human flesh is unique in being that which gives rise to our experience of other material stuff. It is that through which we experience and interact with our world. This cannot be said of other objects. Other useful, unitive theories of the body/mind or 'self' have been proposed by certain schools of psychotherapy, notably modern gestalt psychotherapy.

Another alternative way of explaining how manual practitioners treat people, rather than merely their bodies, would be to propose a transactional psychological element explicit in the manual therapeutic method. If not, any psychological effect would be incidental or in addition to that method, and not inherently attributable to it. Patients are always both soul and body. They are not one or the other in different circumstances. The duality is an illusion.

Clearly, there is a crisis in manual therapy theory. It is sensible to open up the debate by examining what practitioners actually do to patients.

SUMMARY OF MAIN POINTS

This chapter has:

1. drawn attention to certain manual therapeutic models which use energy field theory rather than physiological theory. Such models thereby include psychological aspects of patients' problems

2. described certain of the concepts underlying manual therapy including:
— the notion that mechanical intervention produces physiological effects
— the notion that the body has self-repair attributes
— the application of systems theory to anatomical organisation
— the function and characteristics of muscle
— the intervertebral segment and the treatment of segmental facilitation
— the manipulative treatment of psychological problems
— the effects of massage

3. shown that although these concepts are largely mechanical or physiological in nature, they nevertheless all reveal psychological implications upon close scrutiny

4. defined the kind of touching used in manual therapy interactions as being considered to be purely procedural, technical or instrumental, because of the objectives of the treatment

5. briefly reintroduced and contrasted procedural touching with the more usual type of touching in human life, which can be called *expressive*

6. questioned some manual therapists' claims to be treating the whole person, since the literature describes adequately ministration only to bodily phenomena.

The questions of: whether or not physiological and mechanical models adequately explain the current patient/practitioner encounter in manual therapy and; whether or not manual therapy is inherently emotionally and psychologically significant, have so far been largely put aside; nevertheless they remain entirely open.

Touching is an everyday interpersonal event, usually expressive of the nature of the relationship between parties, and therefore explicitly untechnical, unprocedural. Procedural touch is a specialisation within touching behaviour; it is extremely uncommon when considering touching as a whole. To ignore this fact is to make a error of judgement over what occurs in manual therapy. The emotional connotations of touching need to be explored in order to promote a balanced understanding of events in manual therapy.

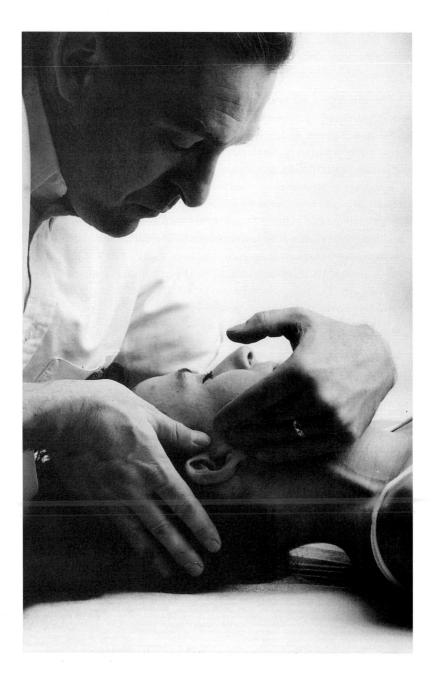

NOTES

[1] It was Aristotle's view that life is expressed in movement, both physical and abstract. Hence the choice of the word 'kinetic' to describe the sum total and variety of effects of human living processes, at least at a physiological or mechanical level.
[2] See for example Rossi (1986), Millenson (1995), Watkins (1997) and the further reading list at the end of the chapter (Further reading: the influence of the mind on the immune system, p 83).

REFERENCES

Angyal A 1981 A logic of systems. In: Emery F E (ed) Systems thinking. Penguin, London, pp 27–40

Boyling J D, Palastanga N (eds) 1994 Grieve's modern manual therapy. Churchill Livingstone, Edinburgh

Bradford S 1965 Role of osteopathic manipulative therapy in emotional disorders: a physiologic hypothesis. Journal of the American Medical Association 64: 484–493

Descartes R 1972 Treatise of man. Translated and edited by Thomas Steele Hall. Harvard University Press, Cambridge, MA, p 113 (Quoted in Leder D 1992 A tale of two bodies. In: The body in medical thought and practice. Philosophy and Medicine Series, Vol. 43. Kluwer Academic Publishers, Dordrecht)

Dunn F 1948 The osteopathic management of psychosomatic problems. Journal of the American Osteopathic Association 48(4): 196–199

Dunn F 1950 Osteopathic concepts in psychiatry. Journal of the American Osteopathic Association 49: 354–357

Dunn F 1952 Altered cervical and thoracic vertebral mechanisms in psychiatric disorders. In: Page L E (ed) 1952 Academy of Applied Osteopathy Yearbook: selected osteopathic papers. Academy of Applied Osteopathy, Carmel, California

Everett T, Dennis M, Ricketts E (eds) 1995 Physiotherapy in mental health. Butterworth Heinemann, Oxford

Gellhorn E 1964 Motion and emotion: the role of proprioception in the physiology and pathology of the emotions. Psychological Review 71(6): 457–472

Haldeman S 1992 (ed) Principles and practice of chiropractic, 2nd edn. Appleton & Lange/Prentice Hall, East Norwalk, Conneticut, ch. 2

Hegna T, Sveram M (eds) 1990 Psychological and psychosomatic problems. Churchill Livingstone, Edinburgh

Hope Robertson R c. 1938 Booklet outlining a proposal for a British osteopathic mental hospital. In: Collins M 1994 Views of the past. British Osteopathic Journal 13: 42–43

Korr I K 1970 The sympathetic nervous system as mediator between the somatic and supportive processes. Post Graduate Institute of Osteopathic Medicine and Surgery, New York

Korr I K 1997 An explication of osteopathic principles. In: Ward R C (ed) Foundations for osteopathic medicine. American Osteopathic Association/Williams & Wilkins, Baltimore, p 7–12

Lederman E 1997 Fundamentals of manual therapy. Churchill Livingstone, Edinburgh

Martinke D J 1991 The philosophy of osteopathic medicine. In: DiGiovanna E L, Schiowitz S (eds) An osteopathic approach to diagnosis and treatment. Lippincott, New York

Millenson J R 1995 Mind matters: psychological medicine in holistic practice. Eastlans Press, Seattle

Patterson M M, Wurster R D 1997 Neurophysiologic system: integration and disintegration. In: Ward R C (ed) Foundations for osteopathic medicine. American Osteopathic Association/Williams and Wilkins, Baltimore
Poon K 1995 Touch and handling. In: Everett T, Dennis M, Ricketts E (eds) Physiotherapy in mental health. Butterworth Heinemann, Oxford, p 94
Roberts A H 1993 The power of non-specific effects in healing: implications for psychosocial and biological treatments. Clinical Psychology Review 13(5): 375–391
Rossi E L 1986 The psychobiology of mind–body healing. Norton, New York
Roxendal G 1990 Physiotherapy as an approach in psychiatric care with emphasis on body awareness therapy. In: Hegna T, Sveram M (eds) Psychological and psychosomatic problems. Churchill Livingstone, Edinburgh, pp 94–95
Schwartz H S (ed) 1973 Mental health and chiropractic — a multidisciplinary approach. Sessions, New York
Schuster C S, Ashburn S S 1980 The process of human development. Little, Brown, Boston
Sheldrake R 1985 A new science of life: the hypothesis of formative causation. Anthony Blond, London, ch. 1
Still A T 1908 Autobiography. Published by the author, Kirksville, MO. Reprinted by the American Academy of Osteopathy, Colorado Springs, 1981
Waagen G, Strang V 1992 Origin and development of traditional chiropractic philosophy. In: Haldeman S (ed) Principles and practice of chiropractic, 2nd edn. Appleton & Lang, East Norwalk, p 33
Ward R C (ed) 1997 Foundations for osteopathic medicine. American Osteopathic Association/Williams and Wilkins, Baltimore, pp 137–151
Watkins A (ed) 1997 Mind–body medicine: a clinician's guide to psychoneuroimmunology. Churchill Livingstone, Edinburgh
Williams J 1986 Physiotherapy is handling. Physiotherapy 72: 66–70
Wittgenstein L 1974 Philosophical investigations. Blackwell, Oxford, p 178
Zusman M 1994 What does manipulation do? The need for basic research. In: Boyling J, Palastanga N (eds) Grieve's modern manual therapy. Churchill Livingstone, Edinburgh, p 657

FURTHER READING: The influence of the mind on the immune system

Berry D S, Pennebaker J W 1993 Nonverbal and verbal emotional expression and health. Psychotherapy and Psychosomatics 59: 11–19
Biselli R, Farrace S, D'Amelio R et al 1993 Influence of stress on lymphocyte subset distribution — a flow cytometric study in young student pilots. Aviation, Space and Environmental Medicine 64: 116–120
Brosschot J F, Benschop R J, Godaert G L R et al 1994 Influence of life stress on immunological reactivity to mild psychological stress. Psychosomatic Medicine 56: 216–224
Cohen S, Tyrrell D A J, Smith A P 1991 Psychological stress and susceptibility to the common cold. New England Journal of Medicine 325: 606–612
Cunningham A J 1995 Pies, levels and languages: why the contribution of mind to health and disease has been underestimated. Advances: The Journal of Mind–Body Health 11(2): 4–11
Dienstbier R A 1989 Arousal and physiological toughness: implications for mental and physical health. Psychological Review 96: 84–100
Dillon K M, Minchoff B 1985–1986 Positive emotional states and enhancement of the immune system. International Journal of Psychiatry in Medicine 15: 13–18
Dreher H 1996 Is there an 'immune power personality'? Advances: The Journal of Mind–Body Health 12(1): 59–62

Dworkin R H, Portenoy R K 1996 Pain and its persistence in herpes zoster. Pain 67: 241–251

Fallowfield L 1996 Psychosocial interventions in cancer. British Medical Journal 311: 1316–1317

Fawzy I, Kemeny M E, Fawzy N W et al 1990 A structured psychiatric intervention for cancer patients: II – changes over time in immunological measures. Archives of General Psychiatry 47: 729–735

Fawzy F I 1994 Immune effects of a short-term intervention for cancer patients. Advances: The Journal of Mind–Body Health 10(4): 32–33

Glaser R, Rice J, Sheridan J et al 1987 Stress-related immune suppression: health implications. Brain, Behavior and Immunity 1: 7–20

Green M L, Green R G, Santoro W 1988 Daily relaxation modifies immunoglobulins and psychophysiologic symptom severity. Biofeedback and Self-Regulation 13: 187–199

Groer M, Mozingo J, Droppleman P et al 1994 Measures of salivary secretory immunoglobulin A and state anxiety after a nursing back rub. Applied Nursing Research 7: 2–6

Jemmott J B, Borysenko J Z, Borysenko M et al 1983 Acadamic stress, power motivation, and decrease in secretion rate of salivary secretory immunoglobulin A. Lancet i (8339): 1400–1402

Kennedy S, Kiecolt-Glaser J K, Glaser R 1998 Immunological consequences of acute and chronic stressors: mediating role of interpersonal relationships. British Journal of Medical Psychology 66: 77–85

Kiecolt-Glaser J K, Fisher L D, Ogrocki P et al 1987 Marital quality, marital disruption, and immune function. Psychosomatic Medicine 49: 13–34

Kiecolt-Glaser J K, Glaser R 1992 Psychoneuroimmunology: can psychological interventions modulate immunity? Journal of Consulting and Clinical Psychology 60: 569–575

Kiecolt-Glaser J K, Marucha P T, Malarkey W B et al 1995 Slowing of wound healing by psychological stress. Lancet 346: 1194–1196

La Perriere A, Tronson G, Antoni M H et al 1994 Exercise and psychoneuroimmunology. Medicine and Science in Sports and Exercise 26: 182–190

Longo D J, Clum G A, Yaeger N J 1988 Psychosocial treatment for recurrent genital herpes. Journal of Consulting and Clinical Psychology 56: 61–66

Lutgendorf S K, Antoni M H, Kumar M et al 1994 Changes in cognitive coping strategies predict EBV-antibody titre change following a stressor disclosure induction. Journal of Psychosomatic Research 38: 63–78

Martin R A, Dobbin J P 1988 Sense of humour, hassles, and immunoglobulin A: evidence for a stress-moderating effect of humour. International Journal of Psychiatry in Medicine 18: 93–105

Rein G, Atkinson M, McCraty R 1995 The physiological and psychological effects of compassion and anger. Journal of Advancement in Medicine 8(2): 87–105

Riley V 1981 Psychoneuroendocrine influences on immunocompetence and neoplasia. Science 212: 1100–1109

Schleifer S J, Keller S E, Camerino M et al 1983 Suppression of lymphocyte stimulation following bereavement. Journal of the American Medical Association 250: 374–377

Toth L A 1995 Sleep, sleep deprivation, and infectious disease: studies in animals. Advances in Neuroimmunology 5: 79–92

Watkins A (ed) 1997 Mind–body medicine: a clinician's guide to psychoneuroimmunology. Churchill Livingstone, Edinburgh

Whitehouse W G, Dinges D F, Orne E C et al 1996 Psychosocial and immune effects of self-hypnosis training for stress management throughout the first semester of medical school. Psychosomatic Medicine 58: 249–263

Wittgenstein 1974 ?

3

The nature of touch

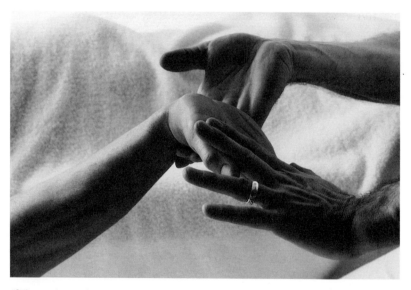

"[The tactile sense] is the fundament of being-in-the-world, for it is the vehicle par excellence by which the person locates himself in space-time."
(Burton & Heller 1964, p 126)

Introduction

This section explores the subject of touch under various headings in order to expose the nature of the relationship between it and emotion. It aims to show that touching is, in an essential way, associated with intimacy. If this is the case, then, since intimacy is emotionally significant, intentional touching is liable to be emotionally significant in essence — however slightly or unconsciously. Such a conclusion would contest the adequacy of the current, purely mechanical rationales underlying manual therapy.

COMMON FORMS OF TOUCH

Interpersonal behaviour involves finding a comfortable balance between making enough contact, while at the same time keeping enough distance. Touching is at the extreme contact end of this range of closeness. The nature of relationships between people can often be worked out by noticing what kinds of touching they participate in.

Communication

The usual way in which touch is considered is as a common but distinct form of self-expression. Touching forms part of the enormous range of bodily movements comprising non-phonetic, non-verbal communication. It is estimated that the major part of communication is non-verbal, eg:

- intonation, emphasis and volume of the voice
- the interaction of voice with ventilation
- non-verbal sounds, cries, sighs, etc.
- movements and postures of the body accompanying different parts of a phrase.

  Communication can be entirely non-phonetic, eg:

- physical closeness
- facial and other bodily postures and movements
- looking
- patting

- incidental touches
- holding
- embracing
- caressing
- sexual contact.

Touching takes up an important position in the spectrum of communication and has certain features worthy of note.

Touch as a short cut

Touching is a unique form of communication. It is profoundly different from language because it can express and communicate emotions and messages which ordinary words cannot. Messages composed of many different ideas can be conveyed in this way — 'wholenesses' of sentiment which would be awkward (or require poetry) to convey verbally. For example, supposing a practitioner attempts verbally to convince a new patient that she is 'safe enough' to be told the 'real' problems; that it is alright for the patient to cry in front of her if she needs to; that she genuinely cares about the patient as a person; that the consultation is completely confidential; that she does not think it childish or silly to be upset; and that she thinks it's acceptable for adults to display vulnerability, etc. Such a monologue would likely appear contrived and clumsy. Carefully considered, a touch on the arm or shoulder could do all this, and therefore speak volumes about the attitude of the practitioner, indicating she is safe and caring. Research shows that touch facilitates self-disclosure and a positive experience of an interpersonal transaction.

The lightest touch on the shoulder of an emotional patient to whom one is addressing questions often dramatically triggers the release of a flood of tears, as the patient's unconscious sense of psychological safety is enhanced. Creating an environment of psychological safety is a moral obligation of any caring practitioner, and it promotes degrees of appropriate trust to be established. There is, however, no guarantee that such sentiments are received in the way they are intended to be and great care should be taken with the exercise of especially non-therapeutic touching.

Truthful touch

Touching, like other forms of non-verbal communication, can be at variance with what is being said. It usually communicates directly an attitude which expresses the toucher's (often subconscious) genuine sentiments. Blondis (1982) notes that a patient can feel a nurse's disgust and disapproval by the way the nurse clears away the bed-pan and cleans the patient up — no matter how hard she may try to force a smile with cheery words.

If there is dislike between people transacting, this will usually be evident in body language and touch forms where these occur. Confusing messages arise if there is incongruity between verbal and non-verbal forms of communication. Such messages, if given off by health care personnel prevent trust being established, and neither patient nor practitioner may understand why.

Telling lies with the body is very difficult because the largest part of any bodily movement is controlled by the unconscious. Only the grossest, coarsest and outermost aspects of any pattern of movements are conscious. Because the unconscious, attitudinal *kinetic* character-istics of actions are common to all persons — at least in the same culture — then non-verbal messages are received as easily and as naturally as they are sent. However, both the giving and receiving of these messages is often on an instinctive level. This is partly why people get feelings about one another when or after interacting with them, without knowing exactly why, or where they came from.

Assertive touch

Touching can also be used to assert one's self-expression — to reinforce and emphasise what is being or has been said. In such cases it is as if verbal communication is not going to get through. Touch as assertion renders the message more intense, profound, important, or raises the level of the sincerity or earnestness of the toucher, by 'holding' the attention of the touched. Physicians and counsellors alike use this — with care — as a reinforcement technique in consultation. A light touch on the arm whilst making a point or giving an important piece of advice acts to anchor the verbal message (Zigmond 1984). A logical extrapolation, or perversion of this facility, is physical violence.

Defensive touch

Touching and the kinaesthetic sense (the sense of one's movement) in general may be used for self-preservation. This is not merely for gross defensive movements, but also more subtle stiffenings and contractions of touching or touched parts of the body, especially where unwelcome species of physical contact are occurring. Such tactile events are important for manual therapists to recognise and interpret accurately since they may indicate a patient's discomfort with, and resistance to, certain forms of touch, that is, intimacy, rather than indicating a painful zone.

To conclude: touching is direct communication because there is no medium through which it happens, as there is for the other four senses. More will be said about this under the analysis of touch as a sense. It is this directness of touching which is, of course, responsible for its being involved in the expression of interpersonal intimacy. This feature contributes to touch being less capable of falseness of expression than other forms of communication.

Movement

Touching can be considered as a species of movement in addition to being a species of expression. It takes a move to execute a touch, and being active — more than being acted upon — is how the business of humanity is done.

It is possible to identify a close friend at 400 metres because her unique movement pattern is imprinted in the memory. Nobody else will ever walk like that, or ever has. Movements (dynamic postures) are individual. They are more unique and identifiable than a fingerprint, and they express character and personality. People move in the way they do because of who they are and what they think. But more importantly movement expresses how and what people feel, the extent of feelings, and especially how long they have been feeling them. This latter aspect is highly significant for bodyworkers and psychotherapists alike, because long-term emotional attitudes alter the form of the body. Movement, being an aspect of physical make-up, is autobiographical. It is the moving picture, where static posture is the single frame photograph.

Touching, then, is a subcategory of this spectrum of movement possibilities, and is likewise idiosyncratic and unique to each person. If a class of student manual therapists is divided into two, and one half is told to lie face down on treatment tables, these 'patients' are quickly able to recognise the individual touches of the members of the class who are roving around the room performing the same techniques upon each recumbent student.

Expressive touch, procedural touch and intimacy

Where touch is used mainly expressively, it expresses feelings, attitudes and sentiments. Where it is used mainly as procedure or technique, it demonstrates knowledge, thought and belief. Here there is a parallel with the two types of behaviour important in the medical consultation — affective (showing empathy and reassurance) and instrumental (providing information, questioning, examining and treating) (Adams 1997). Naturally, there are times when touching is almost pure technique and know-how, for example a subtle and difficult manipulative technique. Likewise there are times when it is almost pure communication, for example holding a grieving friend. Often it is a complex mixture of the two, dependent upon the nature of the relationship and other circumstances.

In ordinary, everyday life, interpersonal touching is almost entirely of the expressive variety, although the degree of cultural variation is huge (Jourard 1966). It is significantly different from procedural or technical touch because it has meaning *in itself*. Whether or not it is ritualistic (hand-shaking for example), it tends to display people's attitudes towards one another. It may convey affiliation, fraternity, affection, care, concern, but sometimes also assertion and aggression. In the main, people tend to touch one another more in proportion as they show simple compassion, or in proportion as they care for each other. Leaving aside for a moment the assertive and aggressive connotations of touching, as a rule, it symbolises/expresses degrees of, and also *is* intimacy.

From a simple touch on the shoulder, to holding hands, a playful punch on the chest, a pinching of the cheek, an arm round the shoulder, full frontal hugging, sexual touching, grabbing or holding or shaking to assert one's message — people are used to being touched in the context of interpersonal relationships.

Sensuality, sexuality and existential fear

In the West and particularly in the UK, where it is an assault to touch another intentionally without permission, the considerable degree of touching taboo which exists serves to emphasise the psychologically significant nature of intimate contact. However, much of this psychological significance is of a sexual nature and has been brought about by the effects of Victorian sexual prudery and the confusion between sexuality and sensuality. Fear of sexuality has led to a decline in the appreciation of sensuality, which is the non-sexual, simple pleasure derived from the normal operation of the senses. Furthermore, the corruption of certain religious notions, such as the association of fleshly things with original sin and uncleanness, has served to worsen the obsession with sex in the presence of sensuality. Whilst it is obvious that intimacy very often has a sexual component, it by no means always has. The difference between compassion and passion allows for 'fraternal' or simple affiliative intimacy, and not necessarily sexual intimacy.

Physical closeness is emotive for another reason — it is existentially challenging. The development of a sense of self depends firstly upon the realisation of what is and what is not self. This realisation involves the conception of boundaries between self and others. The extent to which the sense of physical separateness from others is necessary in order to confer one's self-identity varies considerably. But a degree of this 'safe space' is vital for everyone. Physical intimacy has the capacity to threaten the very separateness and individualness of this self-identity. Because self-identity and the volitional power associated with it are deeply psychological concepts, then physical closeness — especially with relative strangers — carries with it at the very least the possibility of strong existential issues. These usually translate into anxiety or other species of fear.

Tactility is fundamental to all parts of the body, and when experienced interpersonally can suddenly be excruciatingly meaningful, forcing us to sit up and take notice, to feel and face our deepest, most profound feelings and essential needs.

EXPRESSIVE TOUCH IN HEALING

Touch as healing in early life

Expressive touch is the original form of healing. All forms of holding, holding-in-rhythm (rocking), cuddling, rubbing, and unsophisticated massage are healing acts which have their origin in the womb. Health creation in its original form is perfect human wholeness as a state of maintained being, rather than a process of conversion from disease to ease. It is most ideally epitomised by the constant and uninterrupted supply of all needs in utero. After separation of the two beings at birth, the child has to establish its own wholeness. This will take many years and during the initial stages it requires nourishment — tactile nourishment as well as food and other kinds of nourishment. Thus holding, rocking, cuddling, etc, are healing acts of touch. They help to maintain and encourage the development of self-wholeness, self-healing. Hence whatever the cause of distress in a child, the most healing and wholeness-creating act an adult can perform is complete physical care-taking by holding and rocking. Such acts are instinctive, universal and do not have to be taught.

With the gradual evolvement of the individual, this species of healing becomes to some extent less necessary in proportion as the person becomes less frightened, and more autonomous when distressed. In the West, modes of healing have become increasingly more dependant upon sophisticated, knowledge-based systems to the extent that, with few exceptions, bodily ills are no longer treated with touch forms in modern medicine. Instead, remedies are prescribed that apparently depend little or not at all upon interpersonal transactions. (In fact, placebo studies demonstrate considerable variation in outcome with different doctors.) However, it is not at all clear whether touch forms ought to become less frequently used after childhood, and in less sophisticated societies holding and rocking — mothering — are used more frequently in adult, intrafamilial healing and nursing.

The similarities between child-healing touch and 'primitive' healing of adults include an underlying concept of wholeness as opposed to dualism. That is, the instinctive recourse to holding as healing is an implicit recognition of the need to protect, care for and contain the whole being, whether the disturbance to health is physical or emotional. In the case of physical ailments, Western medicine has largely lost interest in the person where there is a machine-mending remedy available.

Infants and young children, having not yet been conditioned to separate physical from emotional distress, react to either in comparable ways, as is evidenced by their frank behavioural characteristics during any kind of distress.[1] In those who express emotion freely, emotional distress is felt in the body, and physical illness produces an emotional reaction.

From instinct to technique

Human beings have been touching each other in times of physical or emotional distress since time began. We touch, draw close and hold people when they are distressed, in despair, deeply unhappy, frightened, when we care and want to look after them, when they are in some sense vulnerable. This is the original and archetypal form of empathy (imaginative projection of one's own consciousness into another being). It is the attempt to lower the level of another's pain by sharing embodiment. In this way the degree of pain may also be somehow shared and thereby lessened.

Instinctive, expressive touch forms, especially holding, remain among the only healing acts available for explicitly emotional distress in adult life. But at the same time, there is currently a rise in the use of touch forms as *techniques*, ostensibly for the treatment of mechanical or functional disorders, as evidenced by the ever growing manipulative therapy professions. In attempting to make good the deficit in touching in medicine as a whole, these professions are utilising the therapeutic modality used most explicitly for healing children (whole person healing) and caring for adults in emotional distress. The common denominator in these latter two is emotion.

The manual therapy disciplines, having arisen in the shadow of Western scientific thought, have attempted to place touch forms in a procedural or technical framework. Holding, rocking, rubbing and stroking touches, which all these therapies embrace, are procedurised versions of expressive touch forms. It is natural, therefore, that members of these professions are fighting hard to ascribe physiological rationales to their techniques in an attempt to become or remain scientifically acceptable. It is also not surprising that 'hard science' has often criticised the manual therapies with the accusation that they work primarily with suggestion or 'placebo'. Since the placebo effect is said to be a function of the patient's feeling more positive with respect to his problem — whether this is conscious or not — it refers to aspects of the elusive 'whole person' healing, or simply healing.

Whilst many manual therapists recognise the pleasure-giving and emotionally satisfying effects of their treatments upon patients, they usually attribute these to factors that do not belong within the theory of their discipline. Since what is and what is not part of the manual therapeutic theory is a matter of definition, these issues remain up for discussion. Practitioners must recognise that their therapeutic pedigree is rooted in primitive and instinctive healing behaviour of the expressive touch variety. This notion alone is capable of significantly informing any debate concerning therapeutic rationale.

The nurse's expressive, healing touch

Unlike medical or paramedical procedures by which the business of medicine is done, the touch of a nurse is by contrast a powerful and famous symbol of compassion. In the high-tech hospital ward or theatre, the rehumanising, non-powerful, *care*-oriented touch of the nurse is balanced against the powerful, vulnerability-creating, *cure*-oriented touch of medical personnel. Sally Gadow (1988) insists that care is the ethical standard by which therapeutic interventions are measured, and should form the context for curative procedures. This is because the exercise of power that curative procedures entail creates a power discrepancy, which always increases the patient's already considerable vulnerability. The exercise of curative power is therefore morally problematic in proportion as it is not demonstrably in the context of care. Since caring touch is expressive in nature, it may form an essential moral context for scientific therapeutic interventions.

The nurse's role, therefore, is of one who counteracts the level of vulnerability conferred upon the patient by the curative processes and associated technical administrations. By the nurse's touch the chasm created by the power discrepancy is crossed, the patient's vulnerability, fear and anxiety are reduced, and the patient is enabled. This happens because, Gadow says, by touch, the nurse exposes her own bodily vulnerability — that of the patient being only too obvious. As this happens a situation of mutuality of vulnerability emerges. The mutuality is also explained in terms of the human-to-human nature of the touch, the fact that there is no power discrepancy inherent in it. It is not a procedure, a human-to-machine technique like all the mechanistic medical touches. Instead it is an expression of empathy, an interpersonal affiliative communication.

When the nurse is not performing a medical procedure (while she is holding the hand of a patient who is having a bone-marrow sample taken, for example), the touching is in the expressive touch category. It evokes the idea of *being-with* and sharing, rather than *doing-unto*. Such an act could quite properly be classified as healing.

In modern medicine, one doesn't heal a patient by touching him or her, one does it by surgery, pharmacology, replacing fluids, etc. Compassionate touching in nursing can be used to enhance the healing effect of the medical intervention — apparently the essential healing act. However, it is classified as an adjunct to medical care. But is nursing merely a finely tuned complement? The possibility that the expressive touch and care of a nurse might be as effective as the powerful and mysterious acts of a doctor in stimulating a patient's self-healing resources remains.

Transferential healing

Adults in modern Western societies touch one another very little. In all countries, the vast majority of touching occurs between babies and infants and their mothers — so much so that the amount of meaningful touching received by adults is a tiny fraction of that received as a baby. Later in this chapter, it is described how an infant's early existential and emotional development is based largely upon its experience of tactile and other bodily feeling events. The memory of infantile states is stored in the adult as a vast data-bank of emotio-tactile and kinaesthetic sensations, instincts and reactions. The significance of this is especially evident during adult-to-adult touching with an inbuilt and considerable discrepancy in power, such as when one allows another to care physically for him. In such cases, for example a manual practitioner–patient relationship with its characteristic forms of touching and holding, regression of the patient to a more infantile state will tend to occur. The physician thereby often becomes endowed with illusory mysterious or omnipotent capabilities. (A baby's parents, of course, *are* endowed with mystery and omnipotence of a very real sort.)

Due to these early influential connotations evoked by touch, it may, in any therapeutic situation, stimulate a parent–child type of transaction on an unconscious level more powerfully than in a relationship where touch is not used. This transference, or projection of attributes and feelings which originate from one's past on to present figures, is used explicitly by many psychotherapeutic disciplines to explore split-off aspects of character. However, there is no precedent for its use in the manual therapies (save those manual techniques utilised by psychotherapeutic models such as biodynamic massage or bioenergetics).

That facet of the placebo effect in healing which is due to the patient's perception of the healer as powerful, mysteriously knowledgeable, capable and caring, could be described as transferential healing. Where such transferential healing is brought about by touching, then it is the expressive and not the procedural component of touch that is causing healing to occur. Research into benign spinal pain syndromes indicates that no current treatment is any better than natural history and the placebo effect (Waddell 1987). Therefore, it is perhaps time that touch-as-placebo was offered a place in the manual therapy rationale melting pot.

GROWTH AND DEVELOPMENT

Touch in utero

Touch is the sense first developed in the fetus, and the skin starts to become sensitive to tactile stimuli after about the seventh week (Frank 1957). Intrauterine experiences comprise kinaesthetic and tactile pressure waves of an infinite variety. Some of the pressure waves later become auditory experiences. Tactile and kinaesthetic experiences range from heartbeat, ventilation and bowel sounds to pressure and shock waves due to the various movements of the mother during gestation. Many of these are constant, regular, rhythmical and phasic. The heartbeats of the fetus and mother will combine, creating waves of resonance and dissonance.

The entire surface of the foetus is in contact with warm amniotic fluid and endometrial tissue at about ambient pressure. It floats freely in neutral buoyancy. There is no air in the lungs or gut, and the sinuses have not developed, hence the fetus is unaware of gravity. The surrounding constant temperature and supply of nutrients directly into the blood also comprise support and protection. This enfolding and supremely comfortable experience of tactility provides complete satiety or total lack of any species of hunger or need. The fetus is held multidirectionally and completely — so much so that it is, in actual fact, at one with the mother. It is the same as her. They are one organism, but they are destined to separate. The experience of a holding, containing tactility therefore originally correlates with oneness, satiety and bliss.

Touch ex-utero

During parturition, the baby is exposed to terrific stroking forces and pressures which are directional and intense. Thus the baby's first experience of physical and physiological strain is associated with tactile experience. It is massaged out of the mother's body extremely powerfully — rejected from its warm all-protective environment. Suddenly the baby experiences the full force of gravity and resistance to movement. The surfaces are hard and unyielding, the light intense, and the ambient temperature mostly colder. Loud, pulsating and recognisable intrauterine noises are replaced by unpredictable, non-rhythmic ones of a different quality.

If the baby is placed immediately on to the warm, yielding, belly of the mother, and covered with her hands, this will ease the transition from unity to duality. The tactile sense enables the maintenance of some contact with 'normal' reality — being at one with the mother. The other immature senses at first flounder and are forcibly stimulated into further development. The physician Frederic Leboyer believes that immediately after birth, this transitional stage of early separation should be as gradual and gentle as possible. He maintains that this is crucial for the infant's ability to form healthy relationships in later life (Leboyer 1975).

Some maintain that 'civilised' mothers' habit of putting babies down rather than carrying them everywhere is responsible for more psychological and social disorder than any other etiological factor. The change from the all-soft, all-touching intrauterine experience to the relatively unyielding and non-touching extrauterine environment should be very gradual. It should be determined by the child's progress and development rather than the mother's wishes (Liedlorf 1986). Winnicott's (1965) theory of maternal holding as facilitating the baby's ability to experience itself fully would concur with this, because the full and positive experience of the self is necessary in order for self to be properly valued.

Touch, therefore, is how life and the ex-utero world is first contacted and even the newborn babe is no stranger to it. The instinctive need for its mother's touch is more powerful than any other. If not satisfied it will lead directly to a sense of utter fear. The mother's touch has been actually part of the baby, not merely a mediating flesh. The child does not know itself as being bounded by borders — it has been borderless. It still primitively 'thinks' it is part of its mother and needs to feel that that reality is still so in order to cope with new experiences. Adults instinctively enfold babies in their arms and bodies. They cover them completely in warmth-providing and touch-providing swaddling, recreating the womb. It will take months of development of bodily experience and projected modes of perception before the world is disclosed as other, and the infant begins to perceive itself as a unity. It is the wholeness of tactile experience, therefore, involving proprioceptive and other kinaesthetic modalities, that gives rise to the experience of the self. At the outset of life, self is a *body-self*; an infant's world is first and foremost a tactile one.

'It is tactility in the new-born infant which is the basic orientation to the mother — that is, to life. The child feels the mother before he sees her. He is uniquely comforted by the mother's closeness, and less so by the blurred image of her face. While nourishment comes from the breast, it is the contact and manipulation of the breast which are as psychologically important as the nourishment itself. In this way the

child preserves the original unity of the two bodies. Separation is more than a psychic fact; it is the actual breaking apart of what was formerly one.' (Burton & Heller 1964)

Norman Autton writes:

'In play mother and child revel in the full indulgence of their sense of touch with all the strength of emotion it can arouse. It is through body contact that they are enfolded in a new dimension of experience; the experience of the world of the other. It is this bodily contact with the other that provides the essential sources of comfort, security, warmth and increasing aptitude for new experiences.' (Autton 1989, p 31)

Mother-touch and touch deprivation

There is not the scope in this work to explore the full development of the infant's sense of self. What is important is that the bonding which occurs between mother and baby is, at first, mediated almost exclusively through touching and holding. The revelation of being valued and loved, of belonging and feeling safe, and being seen as precious, always involves physical contact. This psychophysical attachment has been shown, through a wide variety of theory and study, to be essential for the physical and emotional health of the baby and for the well-being of the subsequent adult (see for example Spitz 1955, Greenwald 1958, Harlow & Zimmermann 1959, Winnicott 1965, Bowlby 1969, Klaus & Kennell 1970, 1976, Montagu 1986). Furthermore, the crucial influences of mother-touch extend to the child's own image of its body (Schilder 1964), its sense of self and the value the child places upon itself.

'Tactile experiences...are highly significant in the development of personality...initial tactile experiences provide the basic orientation to the world and especially the physiological signals which evoke the child's naïve spontaneous responses. These are transformed, elaborated, refined, and increasingly discriminated through gestures, facial expressions, tones of voice and through language, into the most subtle modes of interpersonal communication...These experiences [of early bodily contact] establish the individual's early pattern of intimacy and affection, his first interpersonal relations which apparently persist as a sort of template by which he

establishes and conducts his subsequent interpersonal relations...The baby develops confidence in the world, trust in people, through these early tactile relations which reciprocally establish the meaning of the world for him and also his expectations and feelings toward that world.' (Frank 1957, p 229)

Harlow's monkeys

Through tactile experience the baby experiences life-giving contact and life-giving food, but it is the former that is most nourishing. However, Harlow's experiments with infant monkeys (Harlow & Zimmermann 1959) demonstrated that their need for a soft mother-body exceeded that for body warmth and food:

'a cloth mother and a wire mother were placed in different cubicles attached to the infants' living cage. Eight newborn monkeys were placed in individual cages with the surrogates; for four infant monkeys the cloth mother lactated and the wire mother did not, and for the other four this condition was reversed.' (Harlow & Zimmermann 1959, p 423)

Harlow found that both groups of monkeys showed a distinct preference for the cloth mother and that, compared to contact comfort, 'nursing appeared to play a negligible role' in the development of emotional responsiveness. The monkeys also preferred the cloth mother to a warmed, gauze-covered portion of their cage. Harlow also introduced fear-producing stimuli:

'In spite of abject terror, the infant monkeys, after reaching the cloth mother and rubbing their bodies about hers, rapidly come to lose their fear of the frightening stimuli. Indeed, within a minute or two most of the babies were visually exploring the very thing which so shortly before had seemed an object of evil. The bravest of the babies would actually leave the mother and approach the fearful monsters, under, of course, the protective gaze of their mothers.' (Harlow & Zimmermann 1959, p 423)

Infant monkeys with a wire mother did not cling or embrace her in the presence of the frightening stimuli, whether she lactated or not. They could only hug and rock themselves, vocalise or rub themselves against the side of the cubicle.

Harlow equated the satisfaction gained by the monkeys from soft contact with the provision of love. His experiments: 'indicate the overwhelming importance of contact comfort. The results are so strik-ing as to suggest that the primary function of nursing [suckling] may be that of ensuring frequent and intimate contact between mother and infant.' (Harlow & Zimmermann 1959, p 423). Indeed, adequate contact has been shown to be important for the very survival of neonatal monkeys (van Wagenen 1950).

The detrimental effects of touch deprivation range from the failure to thrive and being vulnerable to various physical disorders, to behav-ioural problems and the inability to relate to other animals socially. Neonatal monkeys which were separated from their mothers a few hours after birth and raised in laboratory conditions showed persis-tent violent emotional behaviour if their blankets covering the wire floor of their cage were removed (Harlow & Zimmermann 1959, p 422).

Infant monkeys need the proximity of their mothers in order to show normal play and curiosity. Kept in isolation from maternal touch-ing, infant monkeys become emotionally and physically isolated and hug and rock themselves and suck their thumbs. They are incapable of play or recreation when introduced to playmates at 6 months. But if such monkeys are returned to their mothers after 6 weeks' separation, they develop normally.

Early touch in humans

The need for touch is perhaps the most basic and innate of human needs. The substituting of surrogates such as blankets and soft toys, and thumb sucking where there is tactile deprivation is commonly observed in human infants (although it is not true that thumb sucking occurs only where there is tactile deprivation).

> 'A baby who is not picked up...lies in his prison crib hour after hour, day after day, with no change or stimulation except when he is fed,...this gradually leads to physical and mental breakdown. This happens because...the 'arousal system' [reticular formation]...must be stimulated regularly to maintain good health. If it is not stimulated deterioration results...' (Berne 1973, p 190)

Failure of an infant to receive continual bodily interaction with its mother at the beginning of its life seriously holds up proper func-tioning of basic physiological processes and leads to personality damage. The whole future learning of the child including speech, cognition and symbolic recognition are all inhibited if he is deprived of tactile experience. This is because tactility is the primary mode both of perceiving and shaping the world and also of communication (Frank 1957, pp. 226–235).

Rene Spitz (1955) investigated the effects of maternal deprivation on very young children. He discovered quite simply that the physical/ emotional tie of the child to its mother is necessary in order for the child to survive:

> 'In the first month of separation, the child shows a weeping, demanding attitude; it is as if the child were reaching out for another person. In the second month the child shows withdrawal, and if you do approach it, it begins to scream; it begins to lose weight and the developmental quotient falls. In the third month of separation the child takes up the characteristic position of lying flat on its belly...it does not want contact with the world; if it is disturbed it screams incessantly. It begins to suffer from severe insomnia, loses weight, becomes a prey to intercurrent infections, becomes accident-prone and has cuts, scratches, bruises and other skin troubles. In the fourth month...the facial expression becomes rigid, screaming ceases and the child begins to wail.' (Spitz 1955, p 105)

Spitz observed severe developmental failure in maternally deprived 4-year-old children. The disorders included considerable weight loss, inability to walk, inability to eat alone with a spoon, inability to dress, inability to use a toilet, inability to talk, and death. Importantly, the hygiene in these institutions was meticulous, the food nutritious, and the medical care of a good standard. Despite this, epidemics were frequent. In one institution the death rate of the maternally deprived was approximately 37%. By contrast, children nursed by their own mothers in a prison nursery in considerably poorer conditions did well, and epidemics were not reported.

These findings disclose the vital importance of maternal contact and its emotionally nutritious properties. Spitz was of the opinion that when a mother is taken away from a child it loses the very foundations of its existence (Spitz 1955, p. 105). It is difficult for adults to realise what the mother means to an infant because an event mimicking maternal deprivation of an infant cannot happen to an adult. The adult's world is vast, but the infant's world consists of its mother. The mother provides and is everything for the child. These emotional riches are conveyed very largely through tactile sensation.

In the early 20th century, mothers in the United Kingdom were advised to keep their babies and children at arm's length for fear of spoiling them — preventing them from responding to discipline — and for fear of infecting them with germs (Autton 1989). This dubious advice may well be responsible for much of the touch-hunger and related emotional problems which we see in our society today, and such advice now seems to have been reversed. It has been recognised that, because a baby is no more than an instinctive creature at that stage, then it should be given all it needs when it needs it in order that it might feel secure and valued. Touch and physical contact in general are therefore now encouraged, as they are believed to be essential for the development of a sense of self-worth and confidence.

Babies receiving more handling develop into children who cry less, smile more, and make fewer demands at 1 year (Autton 1989, p 34). They need fewer verbal commands, and are more inquisitive, linguistically sophisticated and intelligent (Klaus & Kennell 1976, Kennell 1974). Furthermore, a prolonged initial postpartum period of skin-to-skin contact increases the subsequent amount of affection shown to the child (Ainsfield & Lipper 1983).

Touch, love and the body-self

Mother-touch is recognising, appreciating and merging — that is, loving. The emotional significance of tactile contact at this stage of life, therefore, cannot possibly be overemphasised. In our adult body-memories are held every detail of our mothers' caressing, holding and rocking, and the corresponding feelings of security, self-worth, and other goodnesses created by them. These memories exist as emotio-kinaesthetic realities. If they are lacking, this deficiency may contribute to deeply held insecurity, poor self-worth and self-confidence, and subsequent difficulties with communication and the development of healthy relationships. These problems are endemic in the Western world, and, needless to say, detrimental to general health.

The mother's importance is in direct proportion to the helplessness of the infant throughout the first year (Spitz 1955, p 103). The child's helpless phase is one during which it needs to be fed and washed, clothed, and carried from place to place. The manner in which these tactile ministrations are done communicate at once how the parent feels about the child. They also communicate the adult's general character and changing emotions and attitudes. Later these communications are supplemented or replaced by other non-verbal communication and by the use of language. But these latter signs, symbols and communications begin as surrogates for tactile experiences. It is quite clear to an onlooker, from the manner in which a child's genital and anal areas are touched during washing and application of creams, for example, how the parent feels about faeces, genitals and anuses in general (as well as how the parent feels about those of the child in particular). This spectrum of attitudes is communicated directly to the child's unconscious and shapes its feelings about its body and its *self*.

The evidence in this section points to something so obvious that it is often missed; namely that these early bodily experiences are also *self* experiences. It is not merely that they amount to the same thing; they *are* the same thing. And it is not enough to say that such experiences are perceived by the body and thereby affect the mind or soul through neurological connections. They are experiences of the self — the whole, total, unique, individual human self, through and through. Bodily experience *is* psychological experience.

It is true that psychological reality tends to be described in different terms from corporeal reality. Indeed the two may be referred to as different species of reality. But the psychological and the corporeal, whether or not they are ontologically distinct in themselves, do not exist separately but as a merged whole.[2]

The consideration of early human life is perhaps the easiest way to recognise the psychological significance of tactile experience. It is, furthermore, the easiest way to recognise the fact that body and soul are one as the self in everyday life, because of what mother-touch means to the baby. It shows the baby what its self means to its immediate environment, and this shapes what the baby's self means to *itself*. This is a profoundly and intensely psychological/emotional experience. There can be nothing more momentous to the newborn baby or developing infant than the revelation of love and being (or lack of) which certain kinds of touching (or lack of) bring.

ANALYSIS OF TOUCH AS A SENSE

The organ of touch is the whole body

Touch is one of the five senses. The traditional view is that a sensation involves a pathway by which certain kinds of physical information are received. The 'knowledge' is then interpreted using cognitive faculties, and 'coloured' (attributed qualities) using affective faculties. Sensation thus involves an individual's psychological make-up as well as bodily territory. We are familiar with the idea of organs of sense — the eye, ear, olfactory cells, gustatory apparatus, and those parts of the brain associated with the interpretation of these (olfactory lobes, visual cortex, etc). But what is the organ of touch?

The usual response to this question is that it is the skin, because of the extreme sensitivity with which tactile stimulation of the skin's surface is perceived. But this is only part of the story. It is possible to feel oneself breathing, to feel one's heartbeat, even to feel one's guts moving if we lie still and concentrate. But don't we also feel ourselves walking, running, turning over in bed, writing, typing, speaking and laughing? If this is not a tactile or tactual sensation then what is it? Sensation derived from the skin is of a special sort, but we experience our entire bodies tactilely or kinaesthetically. Much of this felt information is unconscious proprioception. It has to be so or else all movements and bodily sensations would impinge upon the consciousness and cloud mental processes to the exclusion of all else. Brief reflection upon the amount, location and types of receptors of tactility reveals that, as a sensation, it is perceived in all parts of the body. A little practical experimentation will demonstrate that the sense in which we feel our bodies move, or merely exist, is the tactile one. (Furthermore, hearing is really a modified form of tactility — where pressure waves of a very high frequency are perceived by specialised apparatus. It is also necessary to touch in order to taste.)

Clearly, then, there is no specific organ of touch — it is the whole body which is felt. This fact, which has escaped scientific attention, renders the sense of touch radically different from its four, now more distantly related cousins.

Touch as object and subject

From this predicate of touch can be deduced another; namely, that to touch oneself is also to be touched by oneself.[3] Rom Harre writes;

> '....touch [of oneself] permits the establishment of a distinction between perceiver and perceived that is wholly within the experiential content of one perceiver. In the sense of touch the body is revealed directly as both the object of perception and the means of perception.' (Harre 1995, p 96)

It is this feature of the sense of touch which is able to point to the body's uniqueness among objects: it is that which discloses itself and the world of other objects. It is an important part of Maurice Merleau-Ponty's phenomenological thesis (Merleau-Ponty 1989) that one who touches himself is conscious of both perceiving and being perceived. Indeed, this concept is pertinent to the question of the relationship between touch and emotional meaning because Merleau-Ponty uses his treatment of the subject of touch and embodiment as significant ground for the understanding of meaning-in-itself.

Similarly, then, to be touched by another is also to touch another, because there is tactile sensation perceived by both persons, both experiencing the touch of another. This attribute is not shared by the other four senses, and in it lies the clue to empathy; we know what a touch will feel like — within certain limitations imposed by peculiar experience — because we touch as if we feel the touch ourselves. If this were not true it would be difficult to learn how to touch according to the demands of circumstances. Furthermore, it obliges the practitioner to use imagination and self-reflection.

Touch is unmediated

The other obvious difference between touch and other senses is its directness. There is no medium needed for touch. Water is needed for tasting, airborne molecules for smelling, light for seeing and pressure waves in a fluid for hearing. It is true that the other senses often require degrees of proximity, especially that of smell and taste, but touch is unmediated and direct, tangible contact. The significance of this is of course that interpersonal touch is inevitably intimate (from the Latin *intimus*, the superlative of *interior*, intrinsic, innermost, characterised by or arising from close union). Touch is the sense which is always associated with close, interpersonal relationships.

The primary status of touch among the five senses

These observations of the peculiar characteristics of touching beg the question: is it wise to regard touch as a sense in the same way as other senses? Is touch really a species of perception equivalent to hearing, vision, and the rest, as it is usually presented?

The seeing, hearing, tasting, and smelling apparatus are immensely sophisticated ways of perceiving our environment. The tactile sense is the least specialised sense in terms of anatomical apparatus because it is the natural and most basic way in which the physical world is experienced. A person's immediate physical world consists of his or her body. Bodies, and bodily interactions (with both animate and inanimate bodies), are experienced with the *felt* sense. This is so fundamental as to be easily missed. Human beings are so busy interpreting symbols that they do not notice their most primordial manner of being — their felt, fleshly being.

From this important idea springs the notion that, instead of touch being just another sense alongside the rest, instead, it should be regarded as that which forms the foundation of our fleshly experience. It should be regarded as that sense upon which other sensations depend for their ultimate meaning. Merleau-Ponty mentions an extraordinary experiment which confirms this observation:

> *'If a subject is made to wear glasses that correct the retinal images [ie invert the image], the whole landscape at first appears unreal and upside down; on the second day of the experiment, the landscape is no longer inverted, but the body is felt to be in an inverted position. From the third to the seventh day, the body progressively rights itself, and finally seems to occupy a normal position, particularly when the subject is active.'*
> (Merleau-Ponty 1989, p 244)

The tactile sense stays the right way up and the vision is made to conform to it, in order to provide for the possibility of normal activity. The significance of this is that vision depends upon kinaestheses and tactility for orientation, due firstly to the bodily experience of gravitational force.[4]

The philosopher Edith Wyschogrod, in her paper 'Empathy and Sympathy as Tactile Encounter' (Wyschogrod 1981) argues that it is not possible to include touch in a generic theory of sensation because touch itself provides the basis for such a theory. The fact that:

■ the entire body is tactilely aware, and that
■ the most primary human encounters are tactile ones,

renders tactile revelations of the environment the most fundamental kind.

'While tactility has often been recognised as presenting unique features, so long as it was taken to be one among the other senses, subject to the same categories of interpretation as sight, hearing and the rest, its idiosyncrasies remained unexplained. For the most part, theories of sense based on the localization of sense experience only functionally differentiates the senses in order to provide a formal structure which would account for all sense acts. But tactility subverts this unitary structure since the body as a whole is the tactile field. The body, with its sensitivity to pressure, temperature and surface qualities, together with its kinaestheses, its felt respiratory movements, its pulse, its hand's capacity for manipulative endeavour, its motility, is the primordial ground of existence as incarnate...Thus the manner in which touch yields the world is the most primordial manner of our apprehension of it. ....If the primordial manner of being of the lived body is to be understood as tactile, then tactility cannot be included under a generic theory of sense but provides its ground.' (Wyschogrod 1981, pp 26, 39)

Far from being a mere certain perceptive mode, instead tactility should be regarded as a profound and primary whole-person experience. That is, experience at the level of essential bodily being. Wyschogrod, like Merleau-Ponty, argues that the tactile sense modifies other senses, perceptive acts and their significance. These controversial conclusions about the nature of touch have been ignored by theoretical manual medicine. They are conclusions that appear worthy of considerable research attention.

Touch is the moving sense

Touch includes the ability to manipulate and make objects, to orientate oneself (one's body) in space. It also includes the ability to be receptive to heat, cold, pressure, surface qualities, and so on. Touch is therefore inseparable from kinaestheses (the perception of bodily tensions and movements) of all kinds (Greek *kinein* to move + *aisthesis* perception). Touch:

> '...*is the sense through which the kinaestheses can at one and the same time become active and also aware of themselves. While many body movements are not at the centre of attention they become focal through tactile sensations.*'

> '*Since touch includes the body's ability to move, it provides the sense of "I can," the ability to do, to push, pull, carry, move, etc.*' (Wyschogrod 1981, p 39)

Because these observations are of such fundamental details, they have been largely taken for granted. The tactile sense includes the moving sense. This important idea has given rise to the theory of muscles and related tissues as sense organs, described briefly below.

Touch and empathy

Edith Wyschogrod's work is even more relevant and exciting because she describes an analogy between touching on the one hand, and empathy and sympathy on the other. The analogy exists because touching is the paradigm of both feeling and being felt (as we have seen above). Touching brings the felt into proximity with the feeler. Empathy and sympathy, too, are 'feeling acts' which bring the self into direct encounter with others. Wyschogrod argues that empathy and sympathy, being both affective, relational acts, can best be understood as experiences of a tactile subject, rather than of a seeing or hearing subject. This is because seeing and hearing are modes of perception which do not require proximity, whereas touch requires contact; the proximity of feeling to what is felt.

The significance of this is that, once again, touch is being used as a fundamental concept upon which the understanding of other human acts depends. This time it is acts of affect or emotion — empathy and sympathy — which are being placed inside the concept of tactile encounter. For all physicians, the facility for empathy is a vital one. The notion that empathy may be best understood and explained by referring to the peculiarities of touching, will be a highly influential insight for all users of manual therapy. If the concept of tactility can be shown to include emotional acts such as empathy, then manual therapy should include affective concepts in its theoretical rationale.

To be embodied as flesh is to be fragile, vulnerable, capable of being damaged (vulnerable: Latin *vulnerabilis* wounding; capable of being wounded). This is an inevitable and intrinsic part of corporeal existence. But it is, quite naturally, this capacity for vulnerability that provides the possibility of a true experience of empathy and sympathy. Therefore these very 'feeling acts' are rooted in bodily fragility; in fleshy, kinaesthetic reality.

Aristotle suggested that the organ of touch, far from being the skin, is the heart. He attempted to account for the fact that there appears to be no obvious sense organ, and his generic theory of sensation requires an organ, a medium and an object. He derived the idea of fleshy vulnerability partly from the notion that flesh, as medium (not sense organ), has imperfect powers of refraction. But also because he noticed that, with sight or sound for example;

> "...we perceive because the medium produces a certain effect upon us, whereas in the perception of objects of touch we are affected not by but along with [my underline] the medium; it is as though a man were struck through his shield where the shock is not first given to the shield and passed on to the man, but the concussion to both is simultaneous."
> (Aristotle 1941, p 43b)

The heart is the symbol of affect, of sentiment, feeling, emotion, attitude, and also of core experience. Because flesh is lived as vulnerability in tactile encounter, as Wyschogrod has shown, then Aristotle is pointing to the intimate relationship between touch, as the most inward sense, and the emotional faculty of the soul. Tactile experiences, then, are heartfelt.

Muscles as sensory organs

Philip Latey (1996) describes muscles as having important functions as sensory organs in their own right. In doing so, he feels that the tactile sense is in fact divisible by five:

1. Skin tactility as ordinarily understood.
2. Outward positional sense and body image, which is highly proprioceptive and movement related. This involves the experience of one's own body-language (non-verbal communication), in external transactions. It is a sense of self-perception and is modified by
— how we imagine others perceiving us, and
— how we want to be perceived.
It is therefore related to the physical, if often unconscious, feelings of pressure in the presence of others.
3. Inward awareness of physical fullness, inner solidity, depth and presence of being. In this category Latey places the more obvious and intense inner sensations we create by, for example, stretching, yawning, laughing, weeping and other sometimes emotionally laden bodily acts. These would include interpersonal transactions such as deep massage and other therapeutic touch, but also feeling tickled, close dancing, holding, hugging, acts of sensuality and sexuality. Emotionally 'moving' experiences of any sort are placed here.
4. Visceral sensation felt to well up in the body from the gut. Included are fear, unease and anxiety, anger and rage, joy and euphoria, pain and loss, but also more cognitive feelings such as despondency, related to weakness and fatigue. The arising of emotion in the viscera is a notion supported by psychotherapists who work with the body, notably biodynamic therapy, biosynthesis, bioenergetics, and gestalt therapy.
5. Finer, more mental sensory functions such as elation and species of pain, depression and misery. Also included are effort, concentration, 'emptiness, numbness, bind, effort, flow, composure' and 'pleasurable drift' (Latey 1997a). Latey includes here experiences that 'light up the brain', or are 'mind-boggling'. He also includes interior discovery and even humour — the experience of language itself as pleasurable.

What is interesting is that Latey tends to fuse expressive motor activity and its emotional content on the one hand, with the sensory perception of it on the other. In category 2 he is equating the emotional experience of being in the presence of others with the sensations given up from the soma. In category 3 he is even more explicitly equating the two, and includes non-transactional expression. In category 4 Latey is now describing frank emotions, yet his context is the sensory function of muscle. He moves from noting that muscular sensation can have emotional content at one end of the scale, to describing emotions as sensory functions at the other. Having made this tactile–kinaesthetic affinity for the emotions, in category 5 he describes events as sensory even as they move from the emotional to the cognitive.

It is by no means clear how the genesis of emotions may be associated with muscular sensation. It is often accepted that emotions arise 'viscerally' and prompt muscular activity as a result. Indeed, emotion is thought to be the motivating faculty (Latin *emovere, e* out + *movere* to move), needing muscular activity to express and eliminate itself. Latey, in insisting on the sensory function of muscle, and on the emotional nature of such sensation, is complicating this notion. It is important to note, however, that his analysis once again clearly demonstrates the merging of affect with the felt sense.

The projecting of sensation into an area of the body — that is, the attributing of sensation to an area as an imaginative act (best exemplified by the phantom limb phenomenon) is one thing. The perception of an actual bodily physiological event by the subjective is another. The distinction between the two remains a matter of unresolved debate. This being the case, then there may be a danger of misleading imprecision if Latey's model is followed without further research. Furthermore, the experience of bodily pleasure such as being massaged, which Latey suggests as being partly a muscular function, is likely to be different from that pleasure derived from reading humorous verse. It is a questionable notion that the latter also arises from musculature, although the reading of humorous verse might itself trigger emotional feelings of bodily pleasure. Latey implies that the perception of one's own mental processes is 'felt' because of sensations generated in the smooth muscle of cerebral vasa nervora, but this may not be an accurate description of events. However, changes have been shown to occur in the physiological characteristics of brain tissue in response to mental acts (Petersen et al 1988, Posner et al 1988).

For the purposes of raising the importance of the body's somatic field as a generator of tactile and kinaesthetic sensory experience, Latey's proposal is very useful. It is also useful as an exercise in merging body/mind discourse.

TOUCH IN LANGUAGE

Emotions and physical sensations are both 'felt'

The most recent edition of the Oxford English Dictionary has six pages devoted to the meanings of touch as noun, verb and noun/verb combination. The significance of this is that the sense of touch, more than any other, provides the experiential and phenomenological ground out of which many subtle ideas, words and phrases have been formed. The meaning and full significance of many symbols depend upon prior tactile experiences (Frank 1957). Such early experiences give the symbol both its meaning and its emotional richness. Edith Wyschogrod's arguments support this thesis and, in the course of exploring structural affinities between empathy, sympathy and touch, she shows that ordinary language is evidence of a link between them:

> *'When we say colloquially, "X is touchy," we mean that X is hypersensitive, vulnerable to injury. When "I am touched by Y's kindness," I mean that Y has compelled me to let down my guard, has drawn close so that I cannot remain indifferent to him. To remain untouched by another is to refuse to engage in a feeling-act which brings to light the other's plight, to refuse to empathise with the other. The active deployment of tactility is expressed in such colloquialisms as "I feel for you," by which we mean my body substitutes for yours, I take on your pain.'* (Wyschogrod 1981, p 40)

Words and phrases used to indicate emotional experience are also commonly used to indicate tactile ones. Gilbert Ryle notices this as he explores mentation and affect in *The Concept of Mind* (1988).

> *'By feelings I refer to the sorts of things which people often describe as thrills, twinges, pangs, throbs, wrenches, itches, prickings, chills, glows, loads, qualms, hankerings, curdlings, sinkings, tensions, gnawings and shocks. Ordinarily, when people report the occurrence of a feeling, they do so in a phrase like "a throb of compassion", "a shock of surprise" or a "thrill of anticipation". It is an important linguistic fact that these names for specific feelings such as "itch", "qualm", and "pang" are also used as names of specific bodily sensations. If someone says that he has just*

felt a twinge, it is proper to ask whether it was a twinge of remorse or of rheumatism, though the word "twinge" is not necessarily being used in quite the same sense in the alternative contexts.' (Ryle 1988, pp 81–82)

Lawrence Frank (1957) also notes the dual affective and tactile use of certain words and concludes that the experience of affect is similar to the experience of tactility. Certain kinds of emotions or feelings are felt in the body as are other more obviously physical bodily sensations.

'...we repeatedly say, "I am touched," or "I feel" which implies both a tactile and an emotional response. Experiences are described as "touching" while many adjectives such as harsh, rough, smooth, tender, warm, cold, painful, imply a tactile sensation or experience even when used to describe non-tactile events. Without prior tactile experiences, these adjectives would carry little meaning.' (Frank 1957, p 214)

The use of 'I feel' demonstrates especially clearly the linguistic unification of affect and tactility in sensation. I may feel angry, miserable, frightened, jealous, joyful, these tight shoes, hungry, the warmth of the sun on my face, your lips on the back of my neck, etc.

Another interesting example of this connection is in the description of posture, itself a word that can be used to mean a physical or attitudinal position. 'Attitude', too, is capable of this dual deployment. Latey (1996) when observing a standing patient, notes the words: stature, standing, stance, attitude, carriage, position, poise, bearing, pose, presence, presentation, impression, impact, outlook, view, manner, footing, situation, place, nature, disposition, bent. All of these can be used both in the description of physical qualities, and also those of character, social and political leaning. These words are not emotional terms, but they are attitudinal tendencies which, Latey and others claim, can be deduced from a person's actual structure. Thus Latey presents the thesis that people manifest in their very flesh, their subjective worlds. This idea is explored further in the sections below on body psychotherapy.

Emotions are physical sensations

So-called emotional pain is felt in the body because true emotions are extraordinarily somatic phenomena. They are not cognitive events despite usually being accompanied by these. Emotions are inner stirrings directed outwardly, associated with profound physiological preparations for action and expression. A little reflection on the experience of joy, anger, fear, shock, misery, jealousy, sexual desire and so on will reveal this fact.

It may seem an obvious point to make, that we feel (emotional) feelings in the body as well as tactile ones. However, confusion arises when psychological language classes feelings such as anger as mental events. Mentation, or thinking, is not by itself an emotional experience. Logic and reasoning processes are not felt, they are simply done 'in the mind', abstracted from the soma. The results of mental processes may give rise to affective phenomena which may arise in the body as feelings. But whereas such feelings are generated in association with the mind's activity, their nature is quite properly to be regarded as bodily. Emotion is so often quite palpably of the same nature as somatic sensation and occurs alongside detectable physiological activity. The relevance of the mind lies in making the associations with past experience, held beliefs and knowledge, so that a person is then moved (emotion = to move out).

Language grows directly, symbolising how life is actually experienced. Therefore, to note that emotional and tactile phenomena are both 'felt' is to make an observation of the human condition at a fundamental level. Such an observation is important evidence of the intimate relationship that exists between emotion and tactile experience.

This is not, of course, the same as saying that tactile experience is also emotional experience. The feeling of my kitchen's flagstones under my bare feet may be a cold, and perhaps unpleasant one on its own. This may be so because such a feeling is biologically necessary in order to point to instinctive or reasonable behaviour that may avoid chilblains — on go my shoes. But if my grandmother's house together with its rich and complex memories and associations was my first and archetypal experience of flagstones underfoot when I was a child, then, if I let myself, I may find this first and foremostly tactile feeling emotionally significant for the rest of my life. Clearly, this is simply to state that memory is sensation-laden. The sense of smell especially is known to be strongly and primitively memory-provoking. But the point is that the nature of the relationship between tactile–kinaesthetic experience and emotional experience is such that much of the latter is contained in the former. How much more emotionally laden, therefore, are memories of interpersonal tactility likely to be.

All sensation is gnostic, that is, it is a primitive form of knowing. From this simple philosophical analysis it is evident that the gnostic faculty of touch has some features which set it apart from the other senses. This analysis therefore raises the importance of touch and touching far above that described by typical physiology textbooks. If there exists a category of tactile experiences which are always actually if not potentially also emotional ones, then it is reasonable to assume that being touched by, and touching another human being fall into it.

SUPPRESSION OF EMOTION IN PROCEDURAL TOUCH

Interpersonal rituals during medical consultations

What happens when procedures or techniques are used to touch people? These touches ought not to be connately emotional exactly because they are technical or non-personal in nature. They are used extensively in manipulative therapy in particular and modern medicine in general. Manual therapists perform techniques upon people's bodies: soft-tissue techniques, thrust techniques, articulation techniques, muscle energy techniques, craniosacral techniques, and so on. Technology springs from the rational mind and knowledge — not from the heart and feelings. We are taught that science and technology are not emotional subjects and to most it would seem absurd if we were to call them such (though, paradoxically, scientific endeavour has always and everywhere incited emotional reactions, and the subject matter of this book is, in a way, one of these emotional reactions against the technological appearance of medicine). Practitioners perform their techniques upon patients — with 'detached minds'. Whereas practitioners treat persons in an atmosphere of respect and caring, patients' bodies are considered in a primarily technological context.

But if touch is so associated with human intimacy and emotional issues as is being claimed here, then what happens to these issues during a visit to the doctor and the ensuing physical examination? These are normally not considered to be emotionally significant events (aside from any fear of what the doctor might find). How is it that physicians of most disciplines are able to touch patients so much and so easily without a second thought, and without emotional issues and feelings surfacing?

Interpersonal relationships of the usual sort take a considerable period of time if they are to become physically intimate, because emotional intimacy is usually a necessary precursor. But health care practitioners can touch a patient's flesh immediately and in virtually any way they those, cutting through the usual rituals and codes of non-therapeutic behaviour. This apparent short-cut, etiquette-waiving phenomenon looks like it might demonstrate just how *un*-intimate the encounter is. However, the truth is that it is really so odd that a degree of physical intimacy can occur sometimes without so much as an introduction that it is presumed to be an impersonal encounter. Are patients forced into an impersonal encounter because of the belief system of modern medicine?

The suppression of emotions

If the evidence presented thus far in this book is sound, that is, that intentional interpersonal touching — especially where both parties concerned are alert and aware — is essentially emotionally significant, then this means that there must be a suppression of the emotive issues surrounding touching and illness during the medical consultation. What doctors and other practitioners actually do when they examine and treat patients would, under normal circumstances, be so intimate that the emotional component is forced into hiding in order to avoid its embarrassing and awkward effects. Patients and practitioners are deluded into thinking the encounter is impersonal — a delusion brought about by two things. Firstly, the various powers of the physician; notably, the implicit permission to examine a patient's body and prescribe as she sees fit. Secondly, the generally held view of the ill person as a failing machine. Self as spiritual–emotional–

corporeal entity has its emotional component prised out of the way, revealing an uncluttered clockwork for scrutiny.

Power

In fact, most people have indeed experienced that undeniably emotional anxiety of a visit to the doctor or other health care practitioner. Patients in a waiting room are by no means in the same emotional state as people on the street. They are apprehensive, nervous, often feeling uneasy and anxious. It is known that patients may appear compliant with practitioners' advice and treatment prescriptions, but that they are by no means compliant once out of the consulting room. Furthermore, patients fresh out of a consultation commonly indicate that they said only a fraction of what they meant to say before they went in. They often consider themselves to be wasting the doctor's time. Anxiety may be experienced:

- about the consultation in general — disclosure and vulnerability
- about the possibility of forthcoming tests
- about being examined.

But it is by no means normally recognised that these feelings are actually relevant to the therapeutic consultation, as they so often are.

The physician's authority, awarded by social standing, expertise in healing and the patient's plea for help, grants permission to touch where otherwise it would be flatly refused. Furthermore, the professional standing of the physician promises an overtly non-personal relationship, despite being implicitly grounded, importantly, in trust. The 'parent–child' nature of the encounter together with its authentic power discrepancy, and the power discrepancy in terms of social status and authority, expertise and mystery, all serve to increase the patient's vulnerability and smallness. And in doing so, they enhance the power and permission of the physician to carry out actions that are undeniably intimate.

The body-machine

If the body is viewed by both parties as a machine which has malfunctioned then it needs to be examined for evidence of the type of malfunction, in order that the latter may be classified, understood and rectified. The modern health care practitioner is coerced into ignoring underlying psychological aetiological factors, because the mechanistic belief system does not include them. Likewise, patients' attitudes to their bodies are often those of onlookers over machines, and of practitioners as mechanics engaged in clever diagnostic and repair processes. Machines and mechanics not being highly emotive notions, why volunteer emotive subjects at the garage? This attitude is reinforced and the emotional suppression encouraged when patients are given mechanical and physiological diagnoses and explanations.

The types of touch used during the physical examination are techniques and procedures for disclosing signs of the malfunction — procedural touch. The examination is a practical, technical and intellectual exercise only. What would, in a non-therapeutic situation, be an intimate and hence emotional encounter, becomes instead one where the patient suppresses or attempts to suppress the emotional associations and responses to the various tactile and close-quarter stimuli. He can do this because he has been educated to believe these stimuli are not emotionally laden. Naturally, the patient may have already deeply suppressed emotional issues; emotional suppression in general is a well-recognised psychological phenomenon. But he will have to work very hard indeed to keep certain of them suppressed during the consultation. They will bubble near the surface as the body-self cries 'this is an intimate encounter, I am exposing my fleshly vulnerability'.

The majority of patients actually strive to present themselves as machines. They may fiercely struggle to divide relevant emotional aspects of distress from their bodily correlates, and even to remove the former from their own awareness. Patients have been taught to behave like machines in the consultation, whereas outside the surgery they may go about their business as whole selves again. Patients and practitioners alike are forced temporarily to convert their experience of touch from the usual expressive sort to the technical sort.

The implicit non-involvement of the psyche in medical touching perpetuates in society the belief that the body is simply a machine. Physical examination by strangers can be permitted only if the normal agenda of intimacy is swept aside. Clearly, many medical procedures would be nigh-on impossible if we did not look upon them as procedures carried out on a dysfunctioning machine, but regarded them instead as essentially invading touches: examination of external genitalia, for example. Most doctors hate doing these things as much as patients hate having them done. They know full well, on some level, there is an acutely embarrassing interaction occurring. But it has to be done, the machine must be checked. But are the unsaid issues important to the medical encounter? Some of them will almost certainly be.

A different scenario

Supposing instead the belief system inherent in our culture were that there is no sense in which body and soul are separated, and that the best therapeutic goals involve the reintegration of the physical with the psychological and the spiritual. In this case the patient would not be under the obligation to park his emotional trailer securely in the waiting room or at home before attempting the consultation.

Imagine a patient approaches the surgery with another episode of intense abdominal pain knowing that it has been brought about by her husband's rejection of her affection and her anticipation of the end of their marriage. She hopes her doctor may suggest some medicine to soothe her physical distress. She knows he will ask her about her relationship and she needs to talk about it. She feels her abdomen contract and feels miserable as she thinks these thoughts. The doctor's caring, sensitive palpation of her abdomen releases a flood of feelings and emotions — including the ache of her unrequited love, and the memory of a loving touch.

A person who, like a small child, feels ill as a self, not merely as a body, will apprehend illness as a whole-person, unitary experience. Such a person is unwell, regardless of where the pain is. This person knows full well that his life's predicaments to date, his feelings and vitality or fatigue all contribute profoundly to his problem. Such a patient would regard a consultation with his doctor and the physical examination as essentially emotive, and would need a person-to-person consultation in the fullest possible sense, not merely a silent, bodily examination, diagnosis and prescription.

But notice what level of maturity this requires of a physician. In order to understand and help a patient deal with her or his important underlying issues surrounding an illness, a phsyician must be aware of the extent to which these feelings are capable of causing confusion if they are not aired in their proper context. Furthermore, the intimacy of the consultation/examination scenario fosters the manifestation of a variety of emotions surrounding intimacy itself, which can confuse the therapeutic relationship unless recognised and carefully contained.

Degrees of suppression

It is clear that there are times when bodily health issues are at least machine-like enough in nature to be considered quite properly without reference to a lot of psychological footnotes (for example the simplest surgical and examination procedures). There are degrees of psychological significance, therefore, when dealing with 'bodily' ailments. But it is doubtful whether ailments are ever totally machine-like in nature, unless flesh is mere clockwork.

If a medical procedure is very unlike a non-medical touch, that is, the more obviously technical it is (or the more the body is removed from the self), the easier it will be for the patient to suppress his psychic associations. This is not always the case, since many people are naturally fearful of invasive procedures, and even technology itself may be distasteful. Although under general anaesthetic the conscious psyche is dramatically uninvolved in surgery, nevertheless the unconscious remains active (and patients, of course, do not remain emotionally impartial to operations or the illnesses that give rise to them). The more the touch resembles or evokes memories of a non-medical, interpersonal encounter, then the more difficult it will be for the patient to suppress relevant issues. In such cases the patient will experience the touches as being of the expressive type, rather than technical. The emotional connotations may be affiliative and compassionate, passionate, sexual, or even violent. Confusing mixtures of memories of maternal touch and sexual touch probably occur most commonly.

It is interesting to consider the development of so-called craniosacral techniques in manual therapy. These are, to all intents and purposes, motionless, and involve extremely light cradling of the head for fairly long periods of time. Such an act resembles a technique so little, if at all, that non-procedural, expressive connotations of being held and cared for are highly likely to arise in the patient's experience during the treatment session.

Fear of diagnosis is another emotional variable — for example inspection of a breast lump for carcinoma. Here there would be the issue of the intimacy of the encounter, especially in view of the area examined, added to the issue of the significance of a positive diagnosis. But this fear is in addition to the underlying emotional agenda and psychological dispositions.

It seems there is a confusion around emotions and medical consultations. On the one hand we are led to believe that a physician is merely examining the body for a mechanical malfunction, in which case emotional issues are irrelevant. On the other hand, patients clearly are markedly emotionally affected by the whole business of the consultation and treatment.

It is not being suggested that modern health care practitioners are unfeeling and uninterested in patients' emotional distress. They all know that patients' characters and perceptions of stress influence presenting problems. However, it is unlikely that practitioners are fully aware of the extent to which their implicit and automatic permission to touch the body contributes to the suppression of relevant emotional details from the consultation. Likewise they may remain unaware of the extent to which the examination of the body — as if it were split off from the person — implicitly trains patients to do the same. How strange it is that the medical encounter seems to dismantle a healthy and whole view of the unwell person, rather than nurture it.

INTERPRETATION, COLLUSION AND THE POSITIVE EXPERIENCE OF TOUCH

Manual procedures in manipulative medicine may appear to be well-boundaried, that is, emotionally safe. Patients can conceive of touch that is non-sexual, non-violent, but nevertheless intimate, patient-centred, and caring. Where techniques are less obviously techniques, and are hence more ambiguous in meaning, verbal explanation during the touching will help to maintain any necessary emotional distance. For example the patient who is having his head held might be told 'I'm putting a leverage through your spine — you probably won't feel much movement'. If the patient were to ask 'what are you doing now?' and was told 'I'm cradling your head', then this might indeed be suddenly more intimate than the patient had imagined. Without the safe, mechanistic explanation, it could suddenly be emotionally unsafe.

On the other hand, should the practitioner invade the patient's experience with a mechanistic interpretation of events? For a patient who is conscious of emotional issues lying at the heart of his problem, the machine-like revelation of leverage through the spine might suggest that the practitioner does not have a deep enough grasp of the problem. It might even render the treatment less effective. Clearly there will be times when verbal collusion with the patient's conception of the problem might result in a more useful initial rapport. Latey (1997:b) favours initial collusion with patients' mechanistic conceptions of their problems in order to establish the therapeutic relationship — even when it is clear that psychological issues are of the utmost importance.

Knowing the patient's conception of how healing occurs might, therefore, be extremely useful for the efficacy of the consultation. This is especially so if the physician is likely to interpret her manoeuvres for the patient; manipulative therapists are particularly likely to do this. Where patients volunteer emotional issues as pertinent to their presenting symptoms, then these concepts too deserve sensitive collusion. In such cases it is important to accept that in those patients who need non-mechanistic healing, the mechanistic rationales are to some extent less relevant.

As a rule patients believe in the body-machine view, and it can sometimes be awkward for them to accept non-technical, whole-person accounts of their problems. Where a diagnosis includes any explicitly emotional subjects, patients may feel the interpretation is inappropriate or painful. The Western psyche is so mechanically minded that practitioners must tread carefully. This is firstly in order to allow the reality of emotional aetiologies gradually to dawn upon their patients for themselves, and secondly because their colleagues' mechanistic rationales may not be sympathetic to these ideas. In practice, it is striking (to this author at least) how grateful and relieved most patients are to be told that it is entirely normal and expected that emotional distress should give rise to bodily disorder. In those patients for whom such interpretations would seem confrontational, collusion — at least initially — is obviously desirable.[5]

Intimate contact that is not overtly technical tends always to be emotionally significant because that is what most emotions are about — intimate relations. In the case of conspicuously technological manipulations it is likely that any emotional response to manipulative therapy will be suppressed in the body-as-machine context of the procedure. In such cases, the emotional potential of treatment is just that. It remains so because having one's body touched by another is emotionally charged. This is due largely to unconscious identification with touching experiences in the patient's bodily tactile memory, in which pleasure will play a large part. We may say that this or that technique is a local-tissue technique only and devoid of meaning, and we may have reasonable arguments upon which this statement rests. Nevertheless a patient may experience our touch (consciously or unconsciously) emotionally, whatever we may say.

It is hoped that, regardless of a patient's past, a positive experience of a practitioner's touch will induce feelings of improved self-image, increased self-worth and well-being. This will occur where touch is caring, sensitive, confident, competent and respectful, and is accompanied by explanations and requests for permission to perform techniques. These positive feelings will generate and reinforce the patient's belief that healing is taking place. This, in turn, will generate bodily physiological healing events.

An emotional and physical experience of being touched therapeutically, that is, an experience of being directly healed, together with:

- confidence in the practitioner's power to heal
- belief that the practitioner knows how to heal
- a feeling that the practitioner desires to heal
  together constitute an extremely potent healing force.

SUMMARY OF MAIN POINTS

This chapter has:

1. looked at touch from the angle of simple interpersonal communication, and indicated some interesting features. For example, touch can convey very complex sentiments; it can convey underlying feelings which are not being expressed verbally; it can promote psychological safety and trust; it can be used for assertion and defence.

2. reiterated the difference between procedural and expressive touch, the former being the sort used especially in intellectual exploration, the latter being the sort used by the 'heart'. The much commoner expressive touch takes part in and indicates degrees and types of interpersonal closeness.

3. exposed expressive touch as the original form of *whole-person* healing, suitable whether the disorder is overtly emotional or physical. The change from the instinctive use of healing touch to its scientific and technical use is described.

4. drawn attention to the capacity for therapeutic touch to facilitate regression and transference.

5. drawn attention to the tactile context of the fetus's world, and to touch as supremely important in influencing the existential, psychological and physical development of the fetus and newborn infant.

6. described the effects on infants of touch deprivation, which vary from poor physical, social and emotional development to failure to thrive and often death.

7. equated maternal touch with the provision of love and life, and shown how early body experiences are experiences of the self. Thus the study of tactility reveals how the mind merges with the body as the self.

8. pondered on the location of the organ of touch and discovered that it is the entire body. As such, touch is out of the ordinary with respect to the other senses and forms the basis of all other sense modes.

9. shown how touch provides the basis for understanding empathy, sympathy and other affiliative 'feeling-acts'. Significantly, these are acts of intimacy, sharing, and mutuality.

10. equated touch with the kinaesthetic sense, which links tactility with ego, intention and the capacity to *do*.

11. described some ways in which muscles can be viewed as important sensory organs in their own right. Because the sensations they provide are either emotionally significant or are the emotions themselves, this theory once again merges tactility with affect.

12. drawn attention to the importance of early tactile experiences for understanding the meaning of many words and phrases (describing a visual experience as 'harsh', for example).

13. shown how many words have a dual tactile and emotional use. For example 'feeling', 'posture' and 'attitude' can be used in physical, anatomical, psychological and emotional contexts.

14. noted that emotions are felt as physical sensations.

15. described how and why patients suppress their emotions during medical consultations. Such emotions may be acutely relevant to the presenting disorder.

16. noted the capacity for collusion with patients' conceptions of the emotional content of their disorders, and why this might be useful.

This chapter has presented evidence for the emotional significance of touching, by pointing to the 'emotional' features of touch itself. Accordingly, the following section looks the other way around and approaches the subject of touch from the position of emotion. If, throughout life, our experiences with intimacy are associated with our primary experiences with touch (Wilson 1982), then psychotherapy, which deals with the emotional effects of abuse of such primary experiences, ought to shed further light on the relationship between touching and intimacy.

If it is true that manual therapy is emotionally significant to varying degrees, then emotional therapy, that is, psychotherapy, is likely to be physically significant to varying degrees. In which case psychotherapy might be effective for similar kinds of problems to those for which patients consult manual therapists. Conversely, manual therapy may be psychotherapeutic in certain instances and in the right setting. This latter belief is held by the many schools of body psychotherapy.

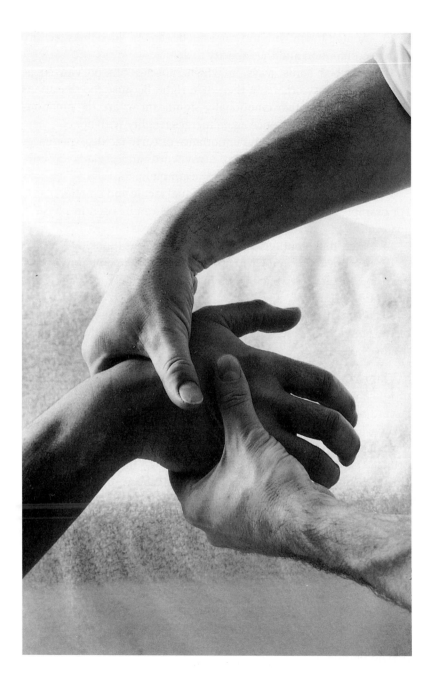

NOTES

[1]The author's son, aged $3\frac{1}{2}$ years, wails 'I don't feel very well' with trembling lower lip, whether he appears to have bitten his tongue, contracted otitis media, feels sick, hungry, tired or cross.

[2]Platonists taught that the soul and the body, although of different worlds, merged to form a soul–body, which had dualistic attributes.

[3]For some women in the late stages of labour, touching the emerging body of the baby is experienced as unpleasant, shocking or unreal. This is because the women expect also to feel themselves being touched. Such expectation is deeply rooted in embodied experience.

[4]The philosopher G. Berkeley (1910) also derives the primary importance of tangibility in interpreting sight.

[5]This, however, might be regarded as an act of dubious ethical status since it contravenes the principle of truth-telling. Encouraging patient autonomy sometimes comes face to face with patient education. Because ethical decisions are a matter of problem solving, it is hoped that in most of these cases the end (a better outcome for all concerned) justifies the means (the initial withholding of certain information).

REFERENCES

Adams N 1997 The psychophysiology of low back pain. Churchill Livingstone, Edinburgh, p 171–172

Ainsfield E, Lipper E 1983 Early contact, social support, and mother–infant bonding. Pediatrics 7(1): 79–83

Aristotle 1941 De anima. In: Ross W D (trans) The basic works of Aristotle. Random House, New York

Autton N 1989 Touch: an exploration. Darton Longman and Todd, London

Berkeley G 1910 Essays towards a new theory of vision. Dent, London

Berne E 1973 Sex in human loving. Penguin, London

Blondis M N 1982 Nonverbal communication with patients: back to the human touch. Wiley, New York

Bowlby J 1969 Attachment. International Psychoanalytical Library, vol. 1, Hogarth Press, London

Burton A, Heller L G 1964 The touching of the body. Psychoanalytical Review 51: 122–134

Frank L 1957 Tactile communication. Genetic Psychology Monographs 56: 211–251

Gadow S 1988 Covenant without cure: letting go and holding on in chronic illness. In: Watson J, Ray M A (eds) The ethics of care and the ethics of cure: synthesis in chronicity. National League for Nursing, New York

Greenwald H 1958 The call girl. Ballantine, New York

Harre R 1995 Physical being. Blackwell, Oxford

Harlow H F, Zimmermann R R 1959 Affectional responses in the infant monkey. Science 130(3373): 421–432

Jourard S M 1966 An exploratory study of body accessibility. British Journal of Social and Clinical Psychology 5: 221–231

Kennell J H 1974 Maternal behaviour one year after early and extended post-partum contact. Developmental Medicine and Child Neurology 16: 172–179

Klaus M H, Kennell J H 1970 Mothers separated from their new-born infants. Pediatric Clinics of North America 17(4): 1015–1022

Klaus M H, Kennell J H 1976 Maternal infant bonding. Mosby, St.Louis

Latey P 1996 Feelings, muscles and movement. Journal of Bodywork and Movement Therapies 1(1): 44–52

Latey P 1997a Feelings, muscles and movement. (Lecture given at osteopathic philosophy conference, Kensington, London)

Latey P 1997b Basic clinical tactics. Journal of Bodywork and Movement Therapies 1(3): 163–172

Leboyer F 1975 Birth without violence. Knopf, New York

Liedlorf J 1986 The continuum concept. Penguin, London

Merleau-Ponty M 1989 Phenomenology of perception. Routledge, London

Montagu A 1986 Touching: the human significance of the skin. Harper & Row, New York

Petersen S E, Fox P T, Posner M I et al 1988 Positron emission tomographic studies of the cortical anatomy of simple-word processing. Nature 331(Feb): 585–589

Posner M I, Petersen S E, Fox P T et al 1988 Localisation of cognitive operations in the human brain. Science 240(4859): 1627–1631

Ryle G 1988 The concept of mind. Penguin, London

Schilder P 1964 The image and appearance of the human body. Wiley, Chichester

Spitz R 1955 The influence of the mother–child relationship, and its disturbances. In: Soddy K (ed) Mental health and infant development, vol. 1. Routledge and Kegan Paul, London

Van Wagenen G 1950 In: Harris E J (ed) 1950 The care and breeding of laboratory animals. Wiley, New York, p 1

Waddell G 1987 A new clinical model for the treatment of low back pain. Spine 12: 632–644

Wilson J 1982 The value of touch in psychotherapy. American Journal of Orthopsychiatry 52(1): 65–72

Winnicott D W 1965 The maturational processes and the facilitating environment. International Psychoanalytical Library, Hogarth Press, London

Wyschogrod E 1981 Empathy and sympathy as tactile encounter. Journal of Medicine and Philosophy 6: 25–43

Zigmond D 1984 Mother, magic or medicine? The psychology of the placebo. British Journal of Holistic Medicine 1(2): 113–119

4

Psychotherapy, touch and the body

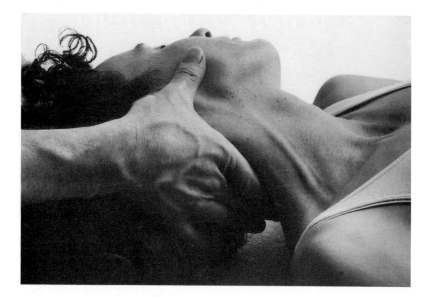

Introduction

This section takes a look at touch and the body from the angle of psychology. The reader is referred to the references and further reading list at the end of the chapter for background reading concerning basic psychology and the place of the body in psychiatry and psychotherapy. The aim of this chapter is to give psychology and emotional subjects a tactile flavour. That is, to show how the study of certain psychological and emotional subjects naturally incorporates the subjects of touch and bodily phenomena.

THE TOUCHING TABOO IN PSYCHOTHERAPY

Touching conveys important interpersonal messages of an intimate nature which are not communicable in other ways (Wilson 1982). It constitutes a primary experience with emotional and trophic effects. Since all of these are important for psychotherapy (Woodmansey 1988), and because many psychotherapists argue that patients often need physical care in order that they may get well, it would be expected that psychotherapists frequently use touch with their patients. But in fact the reverse is true. The vast majority of psychotherapists avoid touching their patients. This has the added effect of perpetuating patients' beliefs that psychological matters do not concern the body, even when such beliefs may not be held by the psychotherapist. Woodmansey, in his article 'Are Psychotherapists out of Touch?' (1988), begins;

> 'Psychotherapists behave as if they had a guilty secret. While the conventional view is that they are forbidden to touch their patients in any significant way, many evidently believe that their patients (or some of them) actually need physical contact — though they tend to provide this furtively and with a feeling of resorting to "poor technique"... Attachment theory logically implies (and experience confirms) that patients who lacked adequate mothering in early life require — like children — actual physical care-giving.'

Since the objective is psychotherapy, then it is the psyche to which the process is addressed. In a cultural and scientific context, which emphasises the intellect and regards it as largely unconnected with the body, it is not surprising that the body has been more or less omitted from the study of psychology. Kepner in his *Body-process: Working with the Body in Psychotherapy* (1993) writes:

> *'Mainstream psychotherapy commonly defines the therapeutic process as working with and correcting mental events and conditions. Tools of the trade have consistently emphasised the "psycho" aspect of therapy — verbalisations, thoughts, ideas, dreams, and the like. Even emotion is viewed as a mental event. Whether the goal is "reduction of psychological conflict" or "improvement of self-image" or "restructuring cognitions", our theories and methods have traditionally attached little importance to body phenomena in the context of psychotherapy.'* (Kepner 1993, p 1)

People tend to consult psychotherapists as a result of abuse of power in their early intimate relationships. This is a précis and a caricature, but it is a true enough observation for these purposes. As the previous chapter has attempted to show, intimate relationships, whether good or bad, are perhaps most profoundly expressed, represented and lived out by various kinds of physical contact.

Abuses of power in early intimate relations often result in a constriction in choice of behaviour in the person's subsequent interpersonal transactions and relationships. The result of this is that the victim of such abuse finds difficulty relating satisfactorily with other persons. Such people often manifest varying types and degrees of anxiety, and maintain a low degree of self-worth and confidence. Psychotherapists assert that one of the simplest yet most profound needs of human beings is to achieve a satisfying and fulfilling intimate relationship with another. Physical closeness is an extremely important if not essential part of this intimacy. Therefore, where there has been an abuse of intimacy in the past (for example inadequate or excessive physical care-giving, or physical care-giving associated with undue assertion, or with aggression, violence, or sexual exploitation), then touching and physical intimacy may still have those traumatic connotations and be directly associated with them in the memory, heart and body of the patient.

The psychotherapist often aims for changes which would result in the patient no longer associating certain aspects of human relationships — namely species of intimacy — with painful, awkward or unpleasant feelings. The success of therapy depends upon the formation of a relationship between the patient and practitioner whereby there is closeness (owing to the nature of the disclosures and the agenda of the mission, so to speak), without sex, violence, or other abuse of power. Such relationships need to be intimate, but with clear boundaries, and founded upon a deep trust.

For some patients, the very fact that the practitioner does not appear to want or need to touch the patient is necessary in order to establish a relationship which is fulfilling but not abusive. In others, the formation of a physically close, but non-sexual, non-violent, non-abusive relationship would theoretically be necessary to facilitate the appropriate changes and growth in the patient's psyche.

The reason why psychotherapists have tended not to touch patients is because of the very real possibility of harming them. Indeed, in terms of the preservation of the patient's safety, the absence of physical contact stands out in orthodox psychotherapist–patient relationships.

The touching of anxious or otherwise psychologically disturbed patients by their therapists, especially whilst exploring issues of past physical, sexual and emotional abuse, might be misinterpreted by such patients as a sexual advance, an invasion of personal space, or as an expression of aggression or hostility (as it might genuinely once have been). Touch might therefore jeopardise the therapeutic relationship, even when it is meant as an expression of empathy, compassion or simple affiliation. The re-creation or symbolisation of the abusive intimate relationship which resulted in the patient's current problem would be so catastrophic for that patient, and is so real a possibility if physical closeness is used carelessly, that psychotherapists have traditionally avoided touching. Kepner (1993) notes:

'Touching and being touched are a fundamental mode of human interaction. In the human interaction of therapy, touch can result in the emergence of unfinished business: one client may have experienced touch as hurtful or intrusive and so *physically organised* himself to expect this kind of tactile contact; another client may have experienced a paucity of tactile contact and so has *physically adjusted* herself to cope with feelings of loss and body hunger for touch...If the body is the part of the self that *has been violated and the reality of the violation itself is denied, then touch threatens to rekindle awareness of having been violated and the need to protect one's boundaries.'* Kepner 1993, p 72–73; [my underline]

Furthermore, psychotherapists know that there is a real possibility that their own needs might be being met if they touch their patients.[1] For example, there is a danger of exploiting power in the same way as patients' parents might have exploited theirs; that is, by using touch as a means to their own ends, as an act of covert self-expression or assertion, rather than as an act which is 'thou-centred' (child or patient-centred). A psychotherapist's desire to be a 'better carer' might result in his wanting to touch a patient at some point during the consultation. Since this is the psychotherapist's need and not the patient's, tradition has urged practitioners to understand their own needs and refrain from seeking to meet them with a patient. Sayers (1996) argues passionately against the use of touch in psychotherapy along these lines, pointing out that: 'It was precisely because the problems bringing women and men to therapy so often involve confusing and collapsing psychological and physical reality that Freud instituted "the talking cure"'. (Sayers 1996, p 120) In writing this, she displays Freud's and her recognition that the physical and the psychological are confused with one another, and merge with one another.

What a paradox it is that the very thing that most powerfully symbolises and indeed *is* intimacy and its emotional connotations — touching — is avoided by those practitioners who intend to cure the problems created by the abuse of such intimacy. On the one hand touch is to be avoided because of this very association. On the other, it is to be recommended in order that the patient experiences and learns to accept non-abusive intimacy without fear. This 'hidden' importance of a possible tactile relation between psychotherapist and patient, 'revealed' by the therapist's usual refusal to participate in it, is what Woodmansey and others have seen as incongruous.

The profound reluctance of psychotherapists to participate in tactile relationships with their patients exposes the importance attached to such relationships in the psychological therapeutic context. It is testimony to the extreme emotional significance of physical closeness, especially when emotional issues are explicitly under scrutiny.

THE USE OF TOUCH IN PSYCHOTHERAPY

In 1982, Jean Wilson wrote: 'Since touch so greatly influences human development, its use as a psychotherapeutic intervention warrants careful attention. Although some writers have considered touch as a therapeutic tool, there are no clear guidelines for its use' (Wilson 1982, p 66). Although some guidelines are now beginning to emerge, the subject remains extremely controversial.

It is likely that beneath this largely laudable restraint from the use of touch and body-work by mainstream psychotherapy lies that same mind/body barrier which has prevented physicians dedicated to alleviating bodily ills from concerning themselves with psychology. Namely, if the psyche and its ailments are not merely separate from, but also of a different character from bodily ills, then it makes as much sense for psychologists to ignore the latter as it does for medics to ignore the former.

However, by no means all schools of psychotherapy now adhere to this view. To the dramatic resurgence of interest in body-work as a generic group[2] has been added a resurgence of psychotherapists attempting to integrate their traditional interest in the patient's psyche with the patient's hitherto neglected soma. These disciplines of body psychotherapy — bioenergetics, biodynamic therapy and biosynthesis and related disciplines — recognise the body as the locus, repository and expressor of emotional events. If the body is the focus of emotional feelings, it must deserve at least some of the therapeutic intervention. Although remaining controversial, the use of touch is also very gradually gaining some acceptance in orthodox psychotherapy.

Hoffman & Gazit (1996) write:

'The use of touch in psychotherapy is a highly sensitive and controversial issue. It goes without saying that physical contact in psychotherapy should be limited to that which is therapeutically supportive and without erotic overtones...Before initiating physical contact, due consideration should be given to the patient's history, values, religious beliefs, dynamics, transference and countertransference elements, timing and its impact on the therapeutic process.'

The authors go on to reject the notion that touch in psychotherapy should only be used when it has been planned in advance and discussed with the client (Hoffman refers to Kertay & Reviere (1993), who suggest that permission to touch should always be sought and intention to touch should always be stated in psychotherapy). They argue the case for spontaneous touch — where 'spontaneous' means neither impulsiveness nor the abandonment of sensitivity and good judgement. Hoffman & Gazit maintain that in certain cases of touch in psychotherapy, the element of spontaneity can be the main factor in creating a positive effect and impact. This is a considerable break with psychotherapeutic tradition.

Osteopathy in psychotherapy

Shaw (1996) makes a brief case for the use of manual therapy in the practice of depth psychotherapy. With a brief literature review, he makes the psychosomatic theoretical link between unsatisfied preverbal needs in the infant and the subsequent development of somatic disorders. He does not believe that problems related to this causal mechanism can be reached by mere verbalisation during psychotherapy since they remain at a preverbal level. Generous supportive touch in the form of manual therapy, being non-verbal, is therefore suggested as an adjunctive mode in psychotherapy. Shaw suggests that during manual therapy the preverbal may be cognised emotionally. This effect is augmented when the patient realises the communicative and expressive significance of certain bodily features, for example, the meaning of neck tension. Because touch challenges feelings which are bodily in nature, it facilitates the re-emergence of aspects of the preverbal self. The preverbal self is essentially emotional and at the same time essentially somatic (see Ch. 3). Therefore both bodily illnesses and their emotional correlates can become more felt, current, and integrated into the wholeness of the self if manual body therapy is used. With adjunctive confrontational depth psychology this integrative effect may be increased.

Shaw, like Randell (1992) before him, describes osteopathic treatment as directly, though often incompletely psychotherapeutic. Osteopathic treatment is likened to Reichian vegetotherapy — which is the use of massage techniques to confront areas of bodily rigidity. Reich maintained that such areas represent psychological conflicts and that physical confrontation in the form of massaging such unrecognised tensions in the physical character would facilitate their becoming more conscious. The osteopath's patient regresses to an infantile state and, using manual treatment as a form of preverbal hypnosis, the practitioner, now a parent figure, holds and supports the patient's traumatised body-self. Holding and rocking allows unconscious, preverbal healing events to occur. Bodily feelings arising during the touching can be profoundly self-communicative, self-informing. They bridge preverbal gulfs, integrating and resolving old emotio-bodily confusions and conflicts. It is as if, in the containing hands of the manual practitioner, the body-self understands itself a little more and can relax and grow in such understanding.

Authors such as Shaw, Randell and especially Latey (1982) make the point that manual therapy's psychotherapeutic potential exists without the need for patients' verbalising their feelings or for deep psychological exploration. This is because recognition of the cause or meaning of long-term muscle contraction ('body-armouring', to use the Reichian term) occurs preverbally. If recognition and integration of these old emotio-somatic conflicts occurs unconsciously, then the need for overt psychotherapeutic dialogue may be obviated.

The production of pleasure by manual therapy is an important part of this theory. The adult patient's symptoms — bodily pain and discomfort — can be seen as a by-product, or even as a necessary creative act of *not feeling* on the part of the infant. This act was once necessary in order to avoid the painful emotional and existential impact of rejection, by the parent, of early infantile needs and desires. Had these needs instead been met and satisfied, they would have produced basic sensual and emotional pleasure. The manual practitioner reintroduces a variety of good feelings back to the patient's bodily experience, including those brought about by the reduction in pain, improvement in bodily ability, holding and rocking, and soothing rhythmic massage. These experiences become frequent and reliable and the patient begins to associate her body with pleasure rather than pain (Shaw 1996). The point is that this is healing a preverbal wound, and not merely satisfying a temporary need for sensual pleasure.

Touching patients has always been known by psychologists to be profoundly emotionally loaded — more so than any other form of interpersonal transaction. It is this fact which led to the near absence of its use in psychoanalysis and psychotherapy. But it is also this fact that has led to a renewed interest in touch as a psychotherapeutic tool in both orthodox and less orthodox schools of psychotherapy. The controversy that such interest is currently inciting confirms the relevance of the subject of touching to psychotherapy.

Furthermore, not just touch, but manual therapy recognisable as standard osteopathic treatment has been acknowledged by some psychologists as being psychotherapeutic — and not merely psychologically significant in some obscure way. Accordingly, such a view includes the recognition of bodily rigidities and discomfort as psychogenic in nature.

MUSCLE DYSFUNCTION

A clinical scenario

Consider the following vignette concerning a patient with some aches and pains who has been examined by a manipulative therapist:

Patient: *'So what have you found; what's wrong with me?'*

Manual therapist: *'Well your upper back seems to be extraordinarily stiff, and I think this is causing your low-back to overwork. Your hips are also unusually tight, as are your pelvic joints, and my feeling is that this, too, throws extra responsibility upon your low back, which is suffering, therefore, from very long-term fatigue. Your low back is rather like the weak link in the chain.'*

Patient: *'Why are these parts of my body so stiff?'*

Manual therapist: *'Well it's difficult to say. It could be the whiplash accident you told me about earlier, together with the fact that you haven't taken any regular exercise for years, plus....some of the stiffness may be inherited, then there's your desk-bound job which hardly encourages mobility, add a little wear and tear superimposed on top....all these add up together to produce the effect.'*

Patient:	*'I see. So what do you suggest?'*
Manual therapist:	*'I suggest we try some manipulation to release the tight, restricted areas, and see if your low back can recover by itself.'*
Patient:	*'What can I do?'*
Manual therapist:	*'You could certainly try some stretching exercises which I'll show you shortly. They should aid the whole process. I'd also like to show you how to try and achieve correct posture when you're working.'*
Patient:	*'OK.'*

The patient received five treatments and felt a little looser after each, but her symptoms seemed to return and there appeared to be no persistent improvement. The patient's general practitioner recommended that she consult the practice counsellor as he felt her problems were caused by 'chronic tension'. The counsellor's explanation for her problems, partly in response to the patient's request for an opinion on the osteopath's findings, gradually emerged over several sessions.

The counsellor said that in his opinion, deep muscle tightness is usually due to tension which is essentially psychological in nature. It is common in everyone to a degree which is highly variable. He agreed that lack of exercise and physical injuries can certainly contribute, but pointed out that he could think of a number of cases of regularly exercising clients, or some with no physically traumatic history who nevertheless felt extremely stiff and tense in certain parts of their bodies. He also made the point that physical injury is psychologically traumatic. 'In my opinion', he said, 'pain such as this is often to do with ongoing, but unrecognised anxieties and depression.'

The counsellor said that the patient's hip restriction may have been set up, appropriately and understandably, at an unconscious level at a time when the patient was experiencing regular emotional and sexual abuse (that this had occurred had emerged during the sessions). He thought the restriction was unlikely to release physically without the patient's 'releasing it on a emotional level'; by recognising and expressing some of the old issues in the counselling relationship. He felt this healing would take time but that there was no reason why it should not occur.

In the counsellor's opinion, freedom of physical expression is dependent to a large extent upon a sense of self-worth and self-confidence. If this is not allowed to develop naturally because of unpleasant formative experiences, then developmental restrictions are placed upon the ability to move, as well as the ability to feel.

The counsellor talked further about the patient's low back ache being perhaps a powerful symbol and reminder of the lack of support she felt from her family and parents. Perhaps, in a sense, she felt unsupported from within. The back pain could be the embodiment of poor support, and the restrictions she felt in her body were also restrictions in her ability to feel certain emotions. This therefore restricted the depth of intimacy she was capable of feeling in her relationships, which, in turn, 'restricted' her well-being in general.

The patient could relate to the counsellor's analysis and queried the diagnosis given by her manipulative therapist. Why she asked, did he not mention long-term tension and anxiety-in-the-body when he was treating her? Why did his analysis seem to depend instead upon non-emotive factors? The counsellor, who was very experienced, said that there were at least two factors. One, manual therapists have traditionally adopted a mechanical view of the body. This has tended to encourage practitioners to pursue mechanical diagnoses — perhaps at the expense of jettisoning more accurate, psychosomatic ones. Two, the unearthing of deeply held emotions, combined with manual therapy, could possibly lead to unhealthy elements in the therapeutic relationship. Even an experienced manual practitioner would need to discharge the patient in order to avoid these, since he was not trained to deal with them. Once such psychological tensions had been unearthed and perhaps explained a little, then it could be that manual treatment might seem less relevant, and that many osteopaths did refer patients to the counsellor for this reason.

The counsellor continued that despite the fact that in his opinion many patients in manual therapy suffer from disorders that contain psychologically generated elements, there was to his knowledge no widely recognised precedent in manual therapy for dealing with them. He acknowledged that many manual practitioners recognise this awkwardness somewhere inside themselves instinctively, but habitually refrain from exploring it. He speculated that most do not want to get involved in psychosomatic diagnoses despite the fact that they may often be the most valid kind. He thought that this was perhaps because some practitioners do not believe in such diagnoses and in any case it is explicit that they deal with physical and mechanical components of disease. The patient continued to see the counsellor weekly.

The causes of muscle dysfunction

The manual practitioner in this example gave an 'extrasomatic' diagnosis, emphasising:

- the passivity of the patient
- the patient's relative impotence to help herself
- the mechanical qualities of the body
- the capacity for the body to be helped by manipulation
- the relative lack of importance of psychological and emotional events.

The psychologist gives a psychosomatic diagnosis emphasising:

- autonomy and activity of the patient
- the patient's capacity to help herself (with the help of the counsellor)
- the emotional qualities of the body
- the capacity of the symptoms to be helped by mental events
- the primacy of psychological and emotional factors.

These are very different approaches, but the patient's primary sign is muscle dysfunction.

There is a large body of psychotherapy literature attending to both the biological significance of psychological events and the notion of working with the body in psychotherapy; for example, Reichian character analysis and technique (Reich 1933), bioenergetics (Lowen 1994), biosynthesis (Boadella 1987), biodynamics (Boyesen 1982, 1985), gestalt bodywork (Perls et al 1951, Kepner 1993). Initially, for manual therapists, the main significance of this perhaps lies in the proposed psychological aetiology of abnormal muscular tone.

Those muscles which are deep determinants of posture, gait, physical attitude, and other personality-dependant movement characteristics are under the control of unconscious elements of the central nervous system (if you are a physiologist) or psyche (if you are a psychologist or psychotherapist). Since the unconscious is that part of the psyche in which psychologists take especial interest, psychology theory ascribes much muscular hypertonia (both short and long term) to psychologically traumatic events. For example, 'repressed infantile traumatised libidinal desires' (Shaw 1996), would result initially in anxiety-driven hypertonia. If such a trauma is repeated or is severe enough, then the problem becomes a long-term one. The persistent emotio-somatic reaction would then produce structural, textural changes in affected muscle tissue rendering it less elastic and less responsive. The initial emotional neural tone would probably gradually disappear as the structural changes replace it. However, it is likely that the memory associated with the emotional cause of the initial high tone, and the emotion itself can, under certain circumstances, be reactivated.

It may in fact be a gross oversimplification to consider muscular dysfunction to be merely an aspect of anxiety or trauma, if it is actually an important feature of character development. Some texts describe the somatic representation of character and personality in great detail, giving examples of specific psychological attitudes together with their corresponding anatomical counterparts (see, for example, Kepner (1993), Lowen (1994), Latey (1982), Keleman (1985), Kurtz & Prestera (1984) and McFarland (1988)).

All this is in stark contrast to textbooks of manual medicine, which, in the main, attribute muscular hypertonia to extrasomatic events. The assumption by manual medicine has been that inappropriately high muscle tone is, in general, a result of insult to the body caused by its mechanical interaction with the environment. That is, it is caused by overuse such as long-term activity of an occupational nature, inappropriately high mechanical loading, or combinations of the two. Such a model sees abnormally high muscle tone as more-or-less independent of psychological constitution. Stress and anxiety are mentioned, though they tend to be seen as less important causes of hypertonia. This is because the tone brought about by current emotional stress is easily palpated as such largely because of the inability of the subject to relax areas of the body which are patently uninjured.

What remains unrecognised is that long term muscular dysfunction can be caused by persistent unconscious psychological tension, which eventually brings about permanent or semi-permanent changes in muscle texture.

Furthermore, it should be pointed out that overtly physical trauma (road accidents, falls, penetration, crush, and impact injury), is itself bound to be psychologically significant (consider, for example, a whiplash patient who can no longer relax in a car and who experiences regular flashbacks and nightmares of the accident: is the cervical hypertonia and perception of pain only organised neurologically at a segmental level, and at the level of local muscle physiology?).

Psychology literature such as that cited above does not consider psychogenic muscle tone to be applicable only to rare cases; these are not abnormal or unusual causes. On the contrary, they are absolutely normal and inevitable, given the eventful nature of life, and the need for people to refrain from reacting with blind emotion to every situation (Baron (1992), in a discussion of phenomenological concepts in the generation of illness, refers to an 'incongruity between intention and achievement'). The terms 'jumpy', 'uptight', 'tense', 'high-strung', 'agitated' are, when applied to a person, psychological descriptions betraying underlying physical characteristics. That is, such a person's characteristic muscular behaviour exposes his level of emotional arousal, or stress. Everyone is familiar with these terms and therefore, at an instinctive level at least, everyone recognises that it is *ordinary* that muscle behaviour should be about personal emotional excitation. The nervous system, after all, is largely set up to move the body and to support its need to move. Psychological and emotional idiosyncrasies colour the qualities of expressive movements, postures and gaits.

Manual practitioners treat psychogenic muscle dysfunction

What is important is that those structures seen as so psychologically significant by body psychotherapists — that is, deep muscular and myofascial tissues[3] — are the very ones in which manipulative therapists also take especial interest.

What are the implications for the manual therapy disciplines of classifying muscular dysfunction as psychogenic? Does this not mean that manual practitioners ought to be conversant with those psychology theories that define abnormal muscle tensions and textures as the physical manifestation of anxiety and 'character armour'? And, if this is so, how should manual medicine incorporate such theories into its own, psychology-free theoretical framework?

Although the notion of psychological causes of muscle tightness, or simply 'tension', is not given great weight in orthodox manual therapeutic theory, it is likely to be well recognised by practitioners. Is the paucity of published attention paid to it because persistent muscle tone — if identified as psychologically induced — may not be a problem for a manual practitioner to solve? This is unlikely since if it were so, then the notion of psychogenic muscle dysfunction would have become problematic for manual medicine long ago. Muscular hypertonia and muscular dysfunction in general would appear to be the bread and butter of most manual practitioners. But just how much muscular hypertonia is psychologically induced, and how much is it induced by 'extrasomatic' events? If long-term, psychologically induced muscle tension exists in everyone to a degree — which experience would appear to suggest — then it is important that manual practitioners set about considering how these patients may be helped.

Theoretical manual medicine ought to research further into the question of psychogenic muscle tone because it is not known if successful treatment of it is achieved by the same mechanisms that resolve 'extrasomatically' generated dysfunction. Practitioners are currently not able to refer to a conceptual framework for understanding how they deal with so-called stress-induced muscle hypertonia. These disorders must surely account for a significant proportion of all muscular hypertonia evaluated by practitioners.

It is inadequate merely to assume that essentially mechanical treatment will resolve psychogenically induced muscular hypertonia without reference either to:

- incidental, non-mechanical effects of the treatment or of the therapeutic relationship, or
- an explicit somatico-psychic treatment sequence rationale.

Neither of these currently exists in accepted standard manipulative therapy theory. Explanations are emerging for understanding how manipulative treatment might help resolve psychologically induced problems. Whether such explanations involve the patient being passive (eg Randell 1992) or active (Lederman 1997, p 121) they involve the primacy of higher centres (the self) and not the mere stimulation of peripheral tissues. Furthermore, if manual therapy can already offer rationales for resolving structural changes in muscle which may have been caused by psychological events early in life (Lederman 1997, p 137),[4] then it needs to develop further insights into what happens to such patients when these problems are treated.

It is a matter for concern that practitioners of health care with such different emphases as manual therapists and counsellors may see the same conditions (ie patients) and give radically different interpretations or diagnoses of the presenting disorder. Why are diagnoses by two experts not the same? Is this difference because the two disciplines see entirely different patient populations? Or is the truth of the situation more likely to be that each discipline overemphasises its own explanation, thereby failing properly to develop adequate and whole insights into departures from health?

Is it possible that manual therapists, steeped in mechanical notions and concepts, are often completely mistaken about the aetiology and nature of their patients' muscular disorders? Or is it more likely that they know full well when there are profoundly psychological reasons for patients' apparently somatic problems (because they recognise different qualities in tissue texture as being generated by different species of aetiological factors), but that they often notice that treatment improves matters? Some practitioners probably even feel that properly applied manipulative treatment given by a respectful and empathic practitioner is able to obviate the need for frank psychological intervention. Certainly the early osteopaths and chiropractors were of this opinion (see Still's (1908) definition of osteopathy; also Hope Robertson c. 1938, Dunn 1948, Bradford 1965, Schwartz 1973).

The implication that manual therapists can help resolve psychologically and emotionally generated bodily disorder deserves much scrutiny and ethical awareness. The implication that psychotherapy can be used to resolve muscular tension of the sort commonly treated by manual practitioners should prompt the latter to re-examine the scope of their theoretical frameworks. The effect of these two notions together is to emphasise the mind–body unity of the self, at the same time as it highlights the confusion created when the two areas are considered separately. Psychological trauma is also trauma to the body. Physical trauma is also trauma to the psyche. Trauma is simply trauma. People — selves — are traumatised, not bodies or psyches. A traumatic event reverberates throughout all aspects of the human being.

THE MERGING OF DISCIPLINES

The question of muscle dysfunction illustrates a wider issue. As physical medicine has become gradually and inevitably impressed with the growing body of evidence pointing to the importance of psychosocial causes of physical disease, so psychologists are becoming impressed with the importance of the physical body in their otherwise mainly intellectual approaches.[5] Both groups are having difficulty in incorporating such knowledge into their theoretical frameworks. As a result of reflection upon such difficulty, certain people in both groups are recognising the need to reformulate the foundations of those frameworks. As a result, newer and wholer definitions of human constitution are being grappled with.

As Kepner (1993) has noted, it is becoming increasingly untenable for health care personnel to see people as other than integral beings. The detached mentalistic trend in psychotherapy which Kepner (1993, p xv) believes created the conditions for the emergence of body-oriented arts and therapies in the 1960s was one extreme of a polarised duality. At the same time the extreme and impersonal scientification of medicine created the conditions necessary for the revival of interest in the *person* in disease, reflected in the rise of holistic theoreticians, alternative therapies and the like.

Therefore one can currently witness a merging, a unification process. On the one hand, health carers with a traditional interest in the body are having to assimilate certain psychological concepts. On the other, carers with a traditional interest in the mind are having to assimilate relevant physical and physiological concepts. One could argue that, were this not occurring, it would be symbolic of theoretical stagnation in the health care disciplines. Such unification is bound gradually to occur. It demonstrates medicine's need to explore and experiment with theoretical frameworks which describe the patient as a unified whole. The overall social question is therefore currently: how and to what extent will there be integration in this merging process? For manual medicine, it is: how will the manipulative professions react and adapt to it?

EMOTIONAL EXPRESSION AND EMOTIONAL ANATOMY

A cursory consideration of the essence of body psychotherapy teachings reveals certain insights necessary for a more realistic approach to manual therapy. These insights can be summarised by the concept 'the inner is expressed in the outer.' This 'law of expression', a Platonic or Aristotelian idea, is a cosmological universal. That is, it is simply one of those principles that appears always and everywhere to be obeyed. The 'inner' refers in this instance to the subjective life of a person. For the purposes of this analysis, it comprises the conceptual and intellectual (the mind), the affective and emotional (the heart), and the volitional, decisive and purposeful (the will). The 'outer' refers to the gross, physical body, including all biochemical and physiological processes.

Inner life expresses itself outwardly. That this is the case is self-evident, and a little reflection will reveal that it could not be otherwise. The law of expression is not merely to restate the obvious fact that thoughts and feelings are expressed in words (or other kinds of noises) and actions. It is also to claim that it is not possible to prevent the inner becoming expressed outwardly, because the inner and outer are merely qualitatively different aspects of the same reality.

For example, for each affective event in the inner life of a person — for each stirring of the affect — there will take place physiological events which are moved *with* that feeling whether the person overtly moves herself or not. The merest thought of moving a part of the body has been shown to produce a detectable neurological readiness in that body system. Similarly, each emotional tone will produce its own shade of physiological arousal. This will be not just in the sympathetico-adrenomedullary system, but throughout the individual's entire, uniquely patterned neuropeptide system. That there is a complex and unique orchestrated wave of neurotransmitter secretion throughout 'appropriate' or 'involved' parts of the body in response to mental and emotional events is now well established.

Thoughts and decisions are to some extent less important here because, although these inform and give rise to actions, they are more removed from the body than emotions are. Purely intellectual functions such as reason and intuition appear to take place at a refined abstract level and produce very little immediate disturbance of the body — though it is true that *belief* itself can trigger profound bodily changes. But subjective events of an emotional nature by definition influence and modify body tissues a great deal and it is therefore of these events that bodyworking practitioners need to be most aware.

Aside from neural tissue, that which is most obviously affected is skeletal muscle, since it makes those gross movements which express feelings. However, visceral smooth muscle, cardiac muscle and secretory tissue are all affected to some extent. Indeed, it is difficult to find evidence of tissue excluded from this effect. Anyone who has experienced the bowel-loosening effect of performance anxiety, for example, will have known the reality of psychophysiological unity. Blushing and sweating are further conspicuous examples. Any and every emotion will affect certain body tissues in certain ways.

A person who is capable of feeling emotions freely and expressing them appropriately will exhibit a body which is supple, elastic and fluid in its movement characteristics. Such a body will always incorporate adequate hormonal and other secretory mechanisms because the alterations in physiological processes which accompany active emotions are purely temporary. Hence each passionate disturbance to the baseline state will resolve as naturally as it arose. Conversely, one who is emotionally out of control or emotionally overcontrolled will exhibit a body with idiosyncratic patterns of disintegrated texture (especially rigidities), mobility, movement and secretory characteristics. With the persistence of unregulated or blocked emotional expression over time, will emerge long-term and even permanent changes in such physical and physiological properties. In this way, the form, textures and motion qualities of a body are shaped. If these changes are severe enough, they will lead to pathophysiological and even pathological events in affected body tissue.

Keleman (1985) writes:

'Life makes shapes. These shapes are part of an organising process that embodies emotions, thoughts and experiences into a structure. This structure, in turn, orders the events of existence...Molecules, cells, organisms, clusters, and colonies are the beginning shapes of life's movement...a person's shape will be moulded by the internal and external experiences of birth, growth, differentiation, relationships, mating, reproducing, working, problem-solving and death. Throughout this process, shape is imprinted by the challenges and stresses of existence. Human shape is marked by love and disappointment.' (p xi)

'Emotional anatomy is layers of skin and muscle, more muscles, organs, more organs, bone, and the invisible layer of hormones, as well as the organization of experience. Anatomical studies tend to depict images that are two-dimensional, thus missing the most important element, emotional life. At the same time, psychology, which is committed to the study of emotion, lacks an anatomical understanding. Without anatomy, emotions do not exist. Feelings have a somatic architecture.' (p xii)

The body-oriented psychology theories rely on the notion that body tissues are shaped in response to both good and bad emotional and cognitive experiences during the formative years. Since the personality and character are formed in exactly the same way, the term 'character structure' (first used by Wilhelm Reich (1933) to denote the part played by muscular 'armouring' in defining aspects of psychological character) is used to describe the bodily form. For psychotherapists interested in the body, its form reveals as much as words do — if not more — of the subject's formative past. It is considered possible to read the book of the body in such a way as to reveal the person's autobiography and also to discover possibilities for creative change.

Psychological causes of form

If the body is identified as the locus of the self, then body tissues form directly in response to and along with their physiological involvement with emotional expression and suppression. Using the language of growth as a metaphor, where emotional expression is free, then body tissues are expansive and vital. Where emotions are bound, so tissues are stunted, constrictive and can appear relatively lifeless.

The biological and biochemical — that is, mechanistic — laws normally considered to govern reproduction, tissue growth, differentiation and other cellular and organismic formative processes are fundamentally inadequate to explain these phenomena even in principle (Sheldrake 1985). They fall far short of explaining the totality of changing tissue qualities throughout life.

There is a missing causative principle from the usual, rather dry accounts of the human person, even in the contemplation of standing posture:

> *'Standing erect is often viewed mechanistically. In these interpretations the human stands erect because of good posture, bones resting upon bones, proper gravitational alignment. The role of human interaction and feeling is dismissed in forming an upright self.'* (Keleman 1985, p 61)

The missing principle is that of emotion.

A race of people forced to live in a series of caves, the ceiling height of which never exceeded their own average height, might be expected to develop a fairly stooped posture with poor development of abdominal muscles. But there are individuals in our own society with similar postural characteristics, whose parents are not morphologically so inclined. Similarly, an individual who works each day with his arms above his head, might be expected to develop hypertrophied deltoid muscles and characteristic changes in his cervical spine. But his working partner may be a different shape altogether.

Environmental demands are thus recognised as being causally formative. If this were not so, there would not be so much attention paid to habitual occupational and recreational posture as being aetiologically significant in physical analysis. Inherited characteristics of form are also recognised, although the debate continues as to the relative contribution of genetics and environment. The influence of the psyche straddles both these areas of inquiry because emotional and psychological aspects of character may be, by present understanding, inherited or acquired. However, the influence of these emotional and psychological attributes and the results of their activities throughout the formative years are not normally considered to be anatomically formative. The mind and its associated emotions have been considered a ghostly presence in the brain, capable of directing certain bodily operations automatically and others with intent. But mind or emotion has not been considered as being influential in the formation of body structure. On the contrary, body structure has always been seen as partly genetically predetermined, and otherwise at the mercy of ruthless environmental pressures and constraints.

Since fleshly matters have always been seen as choiceless mechanics, it is easy to see why the familiar mechanical laws accounting for bodily form and operation are taken for granted. Accordingly, research into the effect of emotional events upon neuroendocrine processes is still in its infancy. After all, if there is no frame of reference suggesting itself as an area of necessary research, then that research is unlikely to be embarked upon. Part of the problem has undoubtedly been that physiological processes have mostly been seen, not as caused by emotion, but as giving rise to emotions. Emotions, therefore, have assumed the status of side effect. It is a relatively new perspective which grants primacy to emotion as physiologically causative.

However, in theory, the pace of physiological discovery has already overturned this attitude. Or at any rate it should have done so in the light of what is known about the physiological effects or expressions of gross emotions. Such understanding is largely in terms of the biochemically steered orientation of body processes in preparation for action (*e-motive* move out) — that is, the familiar 'fight and flight' reaction. The greater part of such information concerns minute-to-minute alterations in the intensity of specific tissue metabolism. However, it is becoming more and more apparent that when such events are unable to be adequately physically expressed or integrated then they give rise to various states of tissue distress. Indeed, it may be that final, physical expression 'expected' by these dedicated physiological preparations is necessary in order that equilibrium can be restored to a sufficient baseline neutrality. From a stable and reliable baseline, further cycles of excitation and withdrawal can then occur. Without such restoration, the cycle of arousal and relaxation becomes disturbed or stuck in some unresolved process. When this happens, both emotional and physiological functioning in general are likely to be compromised because neither the arousal cycle nor the baseline can now operate smoothly.

Research is needed into the effects of long-term activation of these arousal states upon various effector organs. In particular, it is necessary to understand what happens to deep musculature rich in proprioceptive apparatus, and responsible for the uniquely patterned postural configurations of character. It is likely that these muscle systems are as deeply affected by subjective experience as the psyche. This would explain the infinite variations in texture and other physical characteristics palpable by manual practitioners.

The non-expression of emotions poses a problem of complexity for the physiologist, because it introduces the idea of biochemical conflict. For example, an infant's 'biologically normal' rage in response to its parents' denying it something it desires may be met with unsuitably explosive anger by the parent. If the transaction is repeated often enough, the infant's resultant fear will become associated with its expression of rage. That is, the association of the two emotions is then learned — conditioned — in its biochemical as well as in its experiential form. Thus the learning of fear arrives alongside anger, producing a complex orchestration of subtle physical repercussions. Clearly this is a caricature of a description, but only because it is a common occurrence. It is also but one gross example of the continuum of psychological/physical influences endlessly being lived by every person. The individual response to each series of uniquely contextual human interactions will naturally be fine tuned by countless variables. But the psycho-neuro-immuno-endocrino-vasculo-secretomotor-muscular events will inevitably influence the qualities in growing flesh — shape, density, plasticity, reactivity, irritability.

Because of the scientific popularity of mechanical notions of human constitution, there is a paucity of useable models of emotional and psychological human functioning. It would seem that without a psychologico-emotional-somatic map, then a systematic approach to the understanding and assistance of patients is exceedingly difficult to envisage. However, this may not necessarily be so because, as is so often seen, a single trigger can initiate a cascade of healing and transformational events. This is rather like removing a dam in a river; the river knows exactly where to flow — it does not have to be shown.

The constitutional models outlined below and later in this chapter are derived from psychiatric and psychotherapeutic bodies of knowledge. They benefit from their respective attempts to use embryology and tissue organisation — anatomical realities — to inform and evolve psychological understanding.

Keleman's emotio-somatic model

The most explicitly anatomical model of emotional form is that developed by Stanley Keleman in his book *Emotional Anatomy* (1985) which is an exploration of emotional morphology based upon images and diagrams of human form, including visceral form. It is interesting especially for this imagery and also for its use of language, both of which provide an unusually emotive learning experience for the student dry reared on hard science. For example:

> *'Emotions and feelings follow the rules of water. When we brace ourselves for shock or a blow or when we harden to confine pain, our liquid state is like ice. When we melt with love or dissolve into tears, our feeling state is liquid...Feelings and emotions, hormones, bodies, and consciousness all change form and speak in many tongues. Shapes crystallize and liquify. No one is fixed in concrete; rather some processes are ice or bone-like and others are more fluid.'* (p 57)

Keleman's literary style itself constantly crosses mind/body barriers, effectively fusing what are often regarded as separate notions. For this reason his book can feel difficult to understand. This very difficulty may itself demonstrate the degree to which the dualistic conception of persons has become petrified.

Keleman insists that human anatomy is an emotional and kinetic process, distinguished by uprightness and flexibility. These two qualities influence and are influenced by an ongoing emotional story:

> *'Anatomy gives an identity, a specific recognizable shape, and a way of functioning based upon that shape...Shape reflects the nature of individual challenges and how they affect the human organism. Have we stiffened with pride or shrunk with shame? Are we hardened because of deprivation or have we kept safe by collapsing? Does our form indicate a failure to convert feelings into action?'* (p 57)

His model consists of a detailed body plan in terms of tubes, pouches, hollows, compartments and sphincters, stiffenings, pumpings and pulsations. The insults to these forms are in terms of prolongations of aspects of the startle response. The response ideally begins with assertion and moves through a continuum to relaxation, but if the stimulus provoking the response is overwhelming, the end result of the series is defeat. The first part of the response is investigation, challenge, straightening up, becoming more erect — a readiness for action. Next comes rigidification, bracing, hyperextending, pulling back — reflecting fear, anger and attack. Next is flexing forward, closing up, pulling in — self-protective. Lastly comes collapse, falling inward — in order to become invisible or unconscious (Keleman 1985, p 64). Keleman enlarges with considerable sophistication upon these themes and how they are embodied over time as variations and limitations in both morphology and emotional expressivity. He describes four basic general qualities of tissue: rigid, dense, swollen and collapsed. These are artificially separated aspects of the emotional and somatic continuum that is the startle reflex. They represent intensifications and continuations of aspects of the response according to the number, timing, duration, source and severity of threats posed to the individual during his formative life.

The normal startle cycle should ideally be characterised firstly by appropriate contact and finally by full withdrawal. Keleman maintains that there occur combinations of continuations and intensifications of parts of the response; that is, unhealthy deviations from the normal cycle of responsiveness. When this happens the simple startle reflex instead becomes a series of processes permanently affecting and restricting the individual's psyche and soma. For example, an individual may remain in a perpetual state of preparation for action — combat or flight — bracing himself slightly or powerfully, or become weakened and collapsed. These descriptions apply to the psychological and to the full range of physical tissues — muscles, organs and cells. It is important to this theory, as it is to other theories of armouring and somatisation, that responsiveness and flexibility in interpersonal transaction — that is, choice — is diminished or even lost. The person's world of possibilities literally contracts.

Keleman's model is, in part, a psychosomatic expansion and application of the well-known physiological fight and flight response. It argues that the disintegration of this response plays a major part in the process of moulding body shape and tissue qualities according to individual reactions to life trauma. Instead of a temporary, heightened, unstable creative process, the startle reaction becomes a stuck record — unchangeable, dampened, overstable and unfertile. Keleman attempts detailed caricaturing of each stage of the interrupted cycle. He describes characteristic life events psychologically, emotionally and physically, including events in special senses, viscera and body cavities (especially shape and use of the diaphragm), musculature and posture, body wall tissues, gravitational relation, and various physiological activities (eg peristalsis). The emphasis is on the interruption of normal cycles of contact with and withdrawal from challenges, stressors and insults. In normal circumstances the cycles should involve expansion then contraction of body tissues as they are involved in arousal and relaxation. Similarly the welling up and receding of emotions should occur in a flexible array of expressive possibilities. The interruptions of these normal cyclical processes and their subsequent inappropriate unresolved perpetuations are the initial events in both the formation of character, that is, psychological, emotional and physical idiosyncrasies. But they also are involved in the pathogenesis of emotional and physical problems, dysfunction, illness and frank disease.

The idea of the interrupted cycle is a popular theoretical model, implicit in other psychologies, for example gestalt therapy and bioenergetics. Furthermore, the use of the flight/fight response to aid the understanding of physiological aspects of stress and psychosomatic disease in general is, naturally enough, common. Like Latey (1996), Keleman proposes that the options of fight and flight are insufficient as they stand because they fail to account for failure or inability to act satisfactorily. He offers the third option of 'collapse' (similar to Latey's 'lifeless withdrawal').

Bodily shapes and textures are 'the consequences of human attempts to love and be loved...the fulfilment or the betrayal of individual attempts to be human, to have control, to be cooperative' (Keleman 1985, p 149). Furthermore, it is a major part of Keleman's thesis that the bodily shapes and textures are not only autobiographical, but also *give rise* to possibilities for activity, physiology and emotion. They are the effects and also the intending subject. They 'represent the immediate present, how we view the world and try to interact with it for contact, intimacy, and accomplishment'. Constricted, spastic, bloated or weak tissue which has been formed in direct response to environmental pressures, will not merely give rise to pain, discomfort, and unpleasant feelings about the self, but will also determine how the self relates to others:

'If we become rigid, dense or unyielding, we may find ourselves spitefully or fearfully withdrawn. We are unable to reach out or to empathise with others. If we deny our feelings and needs or hide our desires, we may seek out people who also act only out of frustration or who have little interest in their lives.' (Keleman 1985, p 157–158)

Keleman goes on to hint at human interpersonal transactional processes using his anatomico-emotional model. This would be significant for practitioners because a particular kind of transaction would be predicted when, for example, a rigid, controlling practitioner treats a collapsed, depressed patient.

Of necessity, this description of Keleman's theories is a simplification. He notes that combinations of the four major types of structure occur in the same individuals, in different areas and tissues of the body, with left to right and upper body/lower body splits. Different pouches, tubes and body areas may be influenced by the various stages of the startle response, in layers from outer to inner. Each layer may exhibit further compensatory sublayers within itself. Because the overall pattern can therefore be infinitely complicated, it is hoped that there are nevertheless fairly obvious predominant themes which are useful for practitioners.

Emotional anatomy and manual medicine

The significance of this for the practitioner of manual medicine is that palpable qualities of tissue are not merely interesting textural variations in the physical make-up of each person. They are not even only representative of levels of sympathetic tone, or exhaustion. From the aroused states — denseness and rigidity — through to the collapsed states — puffiness, flaccidity and collapse — tissue qualities are pregnant with meaning for each individual. Each is testimony to the individual struggle with lack of acceptance, self-worth and confidence in the face of a hostile formative environment, with which every human being deals.

If Keleman is on the right track, then tissue is emotionally alive and happening, even as it is touched. Manual therapy therefore operates directly in the world of emotions, thoughts and formative processes, however silent or mechanical its apparent practice.

Criticisms of Keleman's model

The two main criticisms aimed at this model are firstly that it is disease centred. That is, the descriptions are exclusively applied to feelings and emotions associated with the startle response and insult and negativity in general. It has nothing to say about the positive side of emotional response, and where this might fit into a general scheme or emotional constitution of man. Secondly, Keleman's model is heavily biologically deterministic, purporting to describe human interaction based largely upon an understanding of biological processes. Whilst this has much to offer in terms of filling an uncomfortable void in our understanding of somatic form, nevertheless, as it stands, it is unclear how it may fit into a more broad map including intellectual, volitional or spiritual aspects of the human condition.

Latey's layers of muscle in postural assessment

Latey (1996) describes four distinct layers of observable posture. The first is what he terms the 'image' posture and this tells us mainly about a person's reaction to being stripped down to underwear and scrutinised in the examination room. Patients often hold themselves in what they believe to be 'correct' body shapes, for example with puffed out chest, held, constricted abdomen and retracted shoulders. A patient may or may not be aware of this degree of presentation of herself for the first part of the examination. Latey refers to this posture as self-conscious. However, the self-consciousness is usually more unconscious (or 'preconscious') than not, in that it can often be diminished if it is drawn to the patient's attention. Latey hints at the point that patients' 'image' postures depend upon who they are presenting themselves to, and this is largely a sexual, and power-discrepancy dynamic. Importantly, then, the image posture is partly a product of the examiner.

The second layer of posture, which Latey terms 'slump' posture, is observed when patients let go of their image, and relax against gravity in their habitual way. It is this posture which gives rise to interpretations such as: shouldering the world's burdens, pillar of society, and so on. This second layer of postural musculature is deeper and longer acting than the first because it is concerned with characteristic antigravity behaviour. Latey notes that despite this first level of relaxation, there are nevertheless often many muscle groups that are still active — in particular expressive areas such as the hands and face.

The third layer of 'residual' posture is that which remains active even when the patient is lying down on the examination table, having become comfortably relaxed. This layer is relatively independent of the effects of gravity. It is largely composed of erector spinae groups of muscle and other paraosteal muscle tissue. These layers often remain extremely hypertonic, comprising a palpable characteristic shape and set of textures. Latey describes these muscles as being the most important for psychophysical study. This is because, as noted above, they are close to involuntary body processes, being controlled by unconscious central nervous systems. Furthermore, these deep spinal tissues are heavily equipped with muscle spindle proprioceptive apparatus and can therefore support and feed back to the process of the unconscious moulding of form. These are the muscles that are most commonly seen to be responsible for felt tenderness, unfelt numbness, and other types of discomfort with which patients typically present. They are those which, as described above, are autobiographical in that they are the physical representations of environmental interactions — both physical and emotional. They correspond with psychological descriptions of character armouring, typical of post-Reichian understanding. This is the layer of musculature that both manipulative practitioners and bodyworking psychotherapists feel they need to come into contact with, for their work to be most efficacious.

Appending his earlier work (Latey 1982), Latey goes on to describe a fourth layer of 'posture' composed of:

'...the respiratory, metabolic and digestive processes which take place within the innermost functioning of our subjective being. It is a compound pattern of breathing, residual postural movement and the peristaltic behaviour of all the involuntary smooth muscles lining the viscera and the vascular matrices of the body. This "inner tube" has its own patterns of stasis, direction, liveliness and eccentric movement also typical for the person.' (Latey 1996, p 47)

Latey goes on to make the connection between this layer and emotional processes, as do bioenergeticists, and other body-based psychotherapeutic models outlined below. He includes fantasy, imagination and 'the depth and breadth of psychological function for the person as a whole' in this layer of posture. These are concepts that are more usually associated with higher, less somatically determined psychological functions. It is doubtful whether this important layer of functioning can be usefully described as posture, but as an aspect of character structure it makes sense. Latey's view could probably be effectively incorporated into Keleman's model (or vice versa).

At this point, it is interesting to note the view of Painter (1987) who insists that layering is a misleading concept when applied to manual therapy, because it leads one to regard the body as an essentially layered structure. Painter argues that much bodywork, when centred upon working through layers, has the effect of merely chasing around tension patterns, which tend to shift around when they are addressed. For example, if superficial outer structures are worked on in order to render them more pliable, perceivable to the consciousness, or even meaningful (interpretable), then tensions in these structures often merely shift from superficial to deep.

Painter insists upon working in a way that views the various depths of the body as being interchangeable. He draws attention to the compensatory reactions of some layers of tissue to others, when layers are considered separately. Painter rejects compartmentalisation and continuously refers to the 'bodymind'. It is not that he fails to recognise, for example, the visceral–emotional layer as an important generator of physiological and psychological processes. It is that he regards the observed reflection and expression of these through all body systems simultaneously as evidence of a kind of immediate, whole interconnectedness. If this is accurate, then body-work requires an analogous approach. Furthermore, having received a non-orthodox background to health care, Painter may be more inclined to a non-fragmented view. Indeed, he may conceptualise a person quite differently from an analytical mind fostered by scientific education. Leder (1990, p 114) has pointed out that the brain, unquestionably the orchestrator of bodily 'intertwinings' (integration) suggestive of an holistic body view, is itself the paradigm of surface-to-depth inter-connection. It is at the core of functions ranging from the intellectual right down to the most visceral. It is placed anatomically at depth and yet it is derived from ectoderm. Therefore, unless it can be shown that the brain integrates the body in an essentially layered way — which is doubtful — then Leder's observation strongly reinforces Painter's view.[6]

Muscle constriction and meaning

Perhaps Latey's most important contribution to the theme of what could be termed 'the presence of mind in the body' lies in his analysis of patterns of muscle constriction and other unhelpful tissue qualities. He considers there to be three major zones of the body: the pelvis; the thorax and abdomen; the head, neck and shoulders. Having described the considerable capacity muscles show for providing sensation (see Ch. 3), Latey goes on to point out that this facility is deployed where other sensation is to be masked.

For example, a common reaction to pain is to clench the fists, writhe, and otherwise contract groups of muscles. This creates powerful sensations capable of interfering with pain gate mechanisms. But the same procedure can be used when feelings of a distinctly emotional nature need to be suppressed. This over-riding of sensation can be at a biological level; for example when a child attempts to prevent urinating by tightening perineal muscles, adductors, psoas and others. It can be at a 'gut' level, as for example, when clenching the abdominal wall to minimise the feeling of fear. It can be at a more respiratory level, as, for example, when stifling spontaneous sobbing by gripping the diaphragm and chest. Or at a verbal level, when, for example, restraining an outburst of loud angry sentiment whilst clenching the muscles of the jaw and neck. Clearly there are overlaps between all these areas, feelings and emotions, but the principles are demonstrated; muscles are used not only to restrict expression, but also to restrict or disallow sensation. Muscles do this by contracting in those ways which amount to a refusal to move expressively, at the same time producing other sensations masking those that were 'intended'.

However, the choicest selection of sensations occurs with expression, not suppression. This is because an emotion produces a need to act. In acting appropriately, the emotional sensation develops, is fully felt, and has meaning:

'The feeling of sadness becomes the act of crying when we allow the sensations to develop naturally into the contractions of the breathing musculature, vocal sobs, and facial expressions of grief. The feeling of longing, when allowed to develop into movement, includes reaching out physically for the loved one.' (Kepner 1993, p 14)

It is important to realise that appropriate emotional events of the kind which occur when one's stability of identity or intent is seriously challenged, should ideally be relatively short lived. They should follow the cyclical series of awareness and crescendo, through to expression (contact) and finally withdrawal and relaxation. By contrast, suppression, by definition, attempts to avoid sensation and therefore involves interruption of the cyclical process. However, muscles are not capable of long-term contraction with impunity. Their physiological health inevitably deteriorates, producing degenerative change in vascularity, collagen content and neurological excitability. This leads to increased density, inflexibility, weakness, tenderness, aching, numbness, tingling, etc. Because muscular activity is essential to emotional expression, the capacity for that expression likewise deteriorates and petrifies.

Using Latey's model (1982, 1996), the pelvis, the site where excretory and genital feelings arise, may find itself becoming a 'fist' of layered muscular contraction. The peculiarities of the muscle behaviour depend upon the derivation and nature of the sensation the individual attempts to suppress. The extent of it depends upon how many layers are recruited to this cause. Latey describes the first layer — the pelvic floor and diaphragm — as being the initial or short-term response. Thereafter, a variety of deep hip rotator/adductor/abductors and abdominal wall muscles are recruited in order to reinforce this for a longer term or more extreme suppression. Because these muscle systems, whilst in a hypertonic state, are incompatible with normal, relaxed and easy locomotor and postural patterns, then further adaptation is necessary in order to create a sufficiently workable synergistic/antagonistic mechanism.

It is obvious that a complex cascade of adaptive responses such as these will play a significant role in the genesis of typical problems with which patients present to manual practitioners. More importantly, the deep layers of this sensation-suppression apparatus (visceral and vascular smooth muscle and deepest skeletal muscle components) will become less competent at registering those sensations indicating dysfunction which normally give rise to compensatory and homeostatic activity. The compensatory and homeostatic activity will therefore fail to occur. This effect will worsen in proportion as the disorder is maintained over a sufficient length of time. The net result is the development of stasis, congestion, irritability, inflammation, susceptibility to infection, and so on, in time perhaps resulting in frank pathology.

Latey's middle fist comprises the 'powerhouse of many intensely emotional movements and feelings' (Latey 1996). It includes the respiratory apparatus including serrati, quadratus, and internal thoracic and abdominal wall muscles. Sensations here include the range of 'gut' feelings, fears and anxieties, but especially discharge of the uncontainable through vomiting, laughing, weeping, yelling and screaming, etc — producing the power behind noise. Latey describes which muscles are involved with masking and suppressing these emotions, together with their aetiological significance in the development of visceral and integumental pathology. The pathogenic mechanisms are thus identical to those of the lower fist.

Latey's examination of the upper fist is a considerably more complicated matter, and the reader is referred to his *The Muscular Manifesto* (Latey 1982), Chaitow's *Palpation Skills* (1996), and 'Feelings, Muscles and Movement' (Latey 1996). The upper fist includes the shoulder girdle, and neck and head. It is involved with refined response and restraint of response to the outside world, and considers the highly complex organisation of neuromuscular systems of the special senses and verbalisation mechanisms. It is an area focusing the more mentally sophisticated blends of feelings of unease, shock and startle, preparedness for conflict, shame, guilt and embarrassment. Other examples are: a feeling of stuckness in the throat, grim determination of the jaw, mental unease expressed in the scalp muscle system, poor range of facial expression, clouding of mentation (with headache), and so on. Again, pathological processes ranging from cardiovascular disease and migraine through to impoverishment of imagination and humour, will have involved, Latey claims, stasis of these anatomical systems and its consequences.

Latey's work attempts to describe in detail a concept which by now will be familiar: abnormal muscular tone can be generated in order to modify or prevent uncomfortable sensorimotor events of a biological, emotional or psychological nature. Because muscles can also prevent the motor expression of appropriate reactions to sensation, then not only the sensory events themselves, but also further ones which would be maximised by full and free expression, are squashed.

Like Keleman, Latey modifies the flight/fight response to include what he claims is the more usual third category — withdrawal. This is characterised by depressed excitability, flaccid muscle tone, and other indicators of lifelessness. Together with deadening of appetites and passions, this withdrawal represents a toning down of responses in general, and is presumably in the face of pressure perceived to be incapable of being healthily integrated. Latey believes this is not merely exhaustion, but is actually an option alongside fight and flight.

For the practitioner of manual medicine, Latey's ideas develop further the idea that biography, personality and emotional vitality are attributes of the living, personable, lived body.

Interpreting postures of body parts

Whereas the psychotherapeutic system known as bioenergetics (Lowen 1976) is probably the most sophisticated discipline associating somatic type with character, postural typing is taken to its extreme form in Kurtz and Prestera's *The Body Reveals* (1984). These authors show how information concerning character and personality are inferred from a detailed examination of standing posture:

> '*A drooping head, slumped shoulders, a caved-in chest, and a slow, burdened gait reflect feelings of weakness and defeat, while a head carried erect, shoulders straight and loose, a chest breathing fully and easily, and a light gait tell of energy and confident promise.*' (Kurtz & Prestera 1984, p 1)

The Body Reveals discusses the influence of gravity upon the upright body. It proposes the notion that the reaction of the body-self to gravity is a reflection of emotional experience. The authors draw especially on bioenergetics, Eastern energetic philosophy, and from the work of Georg Groddeck. They present an extremely detailed piecemeal analysis of the story told by bodily parts, together with interpretations of postural variations. The authors recognise this as partitive analysis, reminding the reader of the necessity to reintegrate and synthesise it with the whole picture of the self. However, they claim the text forms an accurate and useful tool.

Kurtz and Prestera interpret the significance of displacements of mass to the top or to the bottom of the body, or from one side to the other. For example, on examination of one subject:

'... *it becomes completely obvious that two very distinct structures exist within this one individual. These two structures, of course, represent two strongly different trends of his personality.*' (Kurtz & Prestera 1984, p 46)

When speaking of the foot:

'*Through the collapsed arch, more of the bottom of the foot touches the ground. It is an attempt, though a weak one, to experience more of life.*' (Ibid p 48)

And of the knee:

'*The mechanism behind locking of the knee varies with the basic emotional and structural pattern of the individual. [For example, to] keep from being subjugated, stand his ground, maintain a hold on reality, keep the already collapsing structure from falling.*' (Ibid p 53)

And of the pelvis:

'*The unblocked pelvis is able to swing freely forward and backward when walking to allow an easy to-and-fro motion, in contrast to a side-to-side wiggle. In this latter case, the heightened mobility, possibly suggesting greater sexual freedom, may only indicate an increase in local energy charge...[which]...occurs without integration with the rest of the body and is more often associated with an underlying hysteria than with increased sexual appetite or sophistication.*' (Ibid p 58–59)

And of the belly:

'*Overweight...with a heavily padded abdomen, is most often associated with a lack of contact with the belly centre. It is probable that this very lack of contact makes for the individual who constantly eats to fill up.*' (Ibid p 72)

These snapshots merely serve to illustrate particular instances and even then are generalisations in need of the whole-person context in order to provide intelligent insight. Nevertheless *The Body Reveals* is a fascinating collection of observations and revelations comprising a body symbology.

It is important to ask: to what extent are such interpretations reasonable, given the existence of other environmental and genetic causes of bodily form? If they are entirely reasonable then what happens when a practitioner treats patients? Can a practitioner alter bodily form? If so, then if form reflects attitude and emotional life, are these too being altered? If a practitioner is able to free up constricted tissues, is the patient's attitude or emotional stance simultaneously freed? If flesh is the physical form that emotion and attitude take, and in turn informs emotional life, then what are the relevant models that manual practitioners should be using when attempting to understand their interactions?

In general, it is fair to say that the treatises on the anatomical representation of the psyche have not been taken seriously by the scientific community. In fact, they have only received cautious attention within the psychological sciences themselves, whose conceptual framework, like that of medicine, they threaten to disturb. This difficulty in merging is no doubt partly testimony to the inherence of mind–body separation in the orthodox sciences. It is also evidence of the associated barrier in language and concepts which exists between psychology and the physical sciences.

Most people would probably claim to be able to tell when someone is a depressive or an angry sort from that person's body language. Such body language includes a large component of typical standing posture. But it is risky even to generalise about such apparently obvious examples. In the absence of research into the veracity of body symbology, for more subtle symbolic associations between the subjective world and the body, we still have to take an authors' word for it, if they say, for example:

> '*Much of how we deal with reality is expressed in the contact our feet make with the ground. If we are pushovers our feet will show this. They will be inadequate to support us...Rigidity in the foot may reflect rigidity in the person.*' (Kurtz & Prestera 1984, p 48)

Each such assertion by any author must be carefully examined for its plausibility, and this is exceedingly difficult because of the problem of infinite variables described in Chapter 1. But also, and more tiresomely, it is difficult because of the philosophical interruption that exists between describing a person as a pushover, and describing the shape of his foot. Nevertheless, the most constructive line of action would be to accept body symbology as being largely truth, and to follow where this leads in the realms of health care in general.

THEORETICAL ASSUMPTIONS UNDERLYING SOME MODELS OF MIND–BODY

All body-oriented psychotherapy derives from Wilhelm Reich's work, which accordingly deserves a brief summary at this point. Until Reich, the concept of sexual or organismic energy — libido — was considered in rather abstract terms. Although Freud maintained that his theories had their basis in biological science, nevertheless analysis in general paid little attention to the body. Speaking of Reich's departure from Freud's methods, Lowen says:

> 'The laying on of hands constituted an important deviation from traditional analytic practice. In Freudian analysis any physical contact between analyst and patient was strictly forbidden [although Freud's early practice included some stroking of patients' heads]. The analyst sat behind the patient, unseen, and functioned ostensibly as a screen upon which the patient would project his thoughts. He was not completely inactive, since his guttural responses to and spoken interpretations of the patient's expressed ideas constituted an important influence on the patient's thinking. Reich made the analyst a more direct force in the therapeutic proceeding. He sat facing the patient where he could be seen and made physical contact with him when that was necessary or advisable.' (Lowen 1994, p 27–28)

Certainly libidinous energy was not endowed with the explicitly vitalistic–biological properties it was to acquire in post-Reichian theory. Reich was interested in describing libido in as concrete terms as possible, and he decided that the flow of sexual energy could be blocked by actual muscle tension and other physical qualities. Additionally he noticed that his clients' physical styles — postures, movements, voice modulations and patterns of muscle tensing — were serving to prevent their full engagement with the therapist. Their resistance to the attempts by the therapist to interpret their words was thus organised at a bodily level and by no means purely mental, as was currently assumed to be the case. Reich was therefore able to merge the notion of libido with that of resistance to therapy, by connecting them both with physical characteristics (Kepner 1993, p 212).

The following models of body–mind connections suffer from the difficulties referred to at the end of the previous section. Especially confusing is the chronological layering of visceral, muscular, and psychological adaptations. Adaptations may be of different characters and degrees, in different areas of the body, and integrated using a variety of mechanisms. The significance of the adaptations will likewise vary according to time, place and circumstance, and during different interpersonal transactions. For these reasons such models are often accused of being simplistic, but this is not entirely fair since a model is but a symbolic aid to action, and will obviously lack the richness of an authentic interaction.

I am grateful to the authors of *Innovative Therapy in Britain* (Rowan & Dryden 1990) for material summarised and interpreted below concerning Bioenergetics, Biosynthesis and Biodynamic Therapy. They are discussed in this order to correspond with their increasing focus upon the body as the therapeutic subject. The Gestalt approach, the other important body-centred psychotherapeutic school, is then briefly discussed.

Bioenergetics

This model was developed during the 1950s by Alexander Lowen, himself a client and student of Wilhelm Reich. Lowen developed Reich's work considerably and is responsible for the bulk of much bodywork psychotherapy, including that in gestalt therapy.

Bioenergetics draws on Freudian psychoanalytical theory and upon Reichian character structure theory; that is, the relationship between the character and chronic muscular tensions set up in response to frustrated and repressed psychological energy. Accordingly, at its root is the concept of the muscular representation of psychological trauma.

In addition to the psychological problems attributed to trauma, this physical component must be explicitly attended to in the therapeutic relationship for the fullest therapeutic effectiveness. What this boils down to is that if the pattern of muscular tensions expressing psychological disturbance does not change, releasing the tensions in the process, then therapy is incomplete. Probably in recognition of the near-permanent nature of many patterns of long-term muscular fibrosis, Lowen asserted that growth was the key, rather than cure.

The model is vitalistic in addition to being psychosomatic, for it relies upon the notion of the flow of energy throughout the body. The model holds that a free flow of vital energy is necessary for the full capacity for movement, proper colour and temperature, full facial and other bodily expressive characteristics, the experience of pleasure, and the charge and discharge of emotions. Geoffrey Whitfield (1990) summarises the other three major factors in bioenergetic work (aside from energy flow) as character analysis, grounding and breathing. Character analysis includes the observation of typical postural types associated with broad psychological categories. Grounding includes working with exercises to achieve the physical, bodily experience of 'authority-in-the-world'. Attention to breathing is used both as a means to enhance bodily energy and as a means to attain full contact with emotional and somatic feeling. The practitioner will suggest a variety of exercises when working in these areas.

Whitfield further describes, within the person, the four 'layers' containing defences to be worked through, the first two external and the second two internal: one, the presenting problem as described and experienced by the client; two, the character structure of the body of the client which provides armouring against the experience of painful historical emotions; three, a deeper layer storing repressed and unconscious material, and four, the core layer of the vulnerable, needy infant who was injured (Whitfield 1990, p 149). Lowen (1976) summarises these layers as firstly ego, the outermost layer of the personality containing psychic defences such as denial, distrust and blaming, projection (attributing self-attributes to others), rationalisations and intellectualisations. Secondly, the muscular layer of chronic tensions which both support the ego, and also protect against the experience of painful, suppressed emotions. Thirdly, the emotional layer which includes those protected by layer two, for example, rage, fear and despair. Fourthly, the core layer from which the feeling to love and be loved derives. This layer is symbolically and physically represented by the heart — the core (Latin *cor* = heart) of the being. The perception, at this core level, of severe anxiety by the infant begins the process of building defences. Not only do these defences prevent relating to the world with the heart on a freely and appropriately emotional level, but they also protect against actual disturbance of physical heart functioning, threatened by normal, infantile open-hearted relating in the presence of anxiety (Lowen 1976).

Necessarily this is a compressed and subjective version of this model. Of particular significance to manual therapists is the expectation that, under therapy, physical change will occur in terms of appearance and energy: 'It is expected in bioenergetic therapy that there will be significant physical alteration in the bodies of clients because of the recognition of and work on the musculature and posture of the clients' (Rowan & Dryden 1990, p 149). Whitfield describes some aspects of bioenergetic growth during therapy in a case study:

> *'She found that her body could be a reservoir of support and good feelings for herself. She did not have to be tense and ill with psychosomatic ailments. She found a suppleness as she discovered the energy and vitality in her body. That discovery of the harmony was the beginning of a new appreciation of herself which could be rediscovered each day as she left behind the past struggles within her body.'*
> (Whitfield 1990, p 152)

Biosynthesis

David Boadella developed this form of body psychotherapy in the early 1970s. He had worked first with Reichian somatic techniques, and later with bioenergetics and biodynamic psychology (see below). Other influences include Stanley Keleman and Frank Lake. In the understanding of health and illness, biosynthesis derives both from an appreciation of embryology, and from an acceptance of the concept of the non-physical subtle body, which is the energetic regulator of the physical body and its processes. The conceptual layering described by Whitfield and Lowen above is more-or-less adhered to in biosynthesis.

The first two layers are, however, jointly identified to form a three-fold structure. The theory is both very unorthodox and more complicated than bioenergetics.

According to this model, energy from the subtle body differentiates in utero, corresponding with the differentiation of body tissue into the three layers of ectoderm, mesoderm and endoderm. In these tissues the free flow of energy is disintegrated as the armouring process of constructing defences takes place in response to 'the clash between human needs and the 'civilizing' process [which] breaks up the unity of the organism' (Boadella 1990, p 160). It is explicit that the armouring process can take place in utero, immediately postnatally, and during the first few years of life. Disintegration within the fetal subsystems leads to both disruption in physiological terms, between and within the subsystems, and also in psychic terms.

In biosynthesis, the endoderm, comprising the gastrointestinal tract and lungs, is associated with feeling and emotion in general. The mesoderm, comprising bone, muscle and blood, is associated with activity and movement. The ectoderm, comprising skin, special senses and central and peripheral nervous system, is associated with perception and understanding. Consequently, the effect of disorganisation between the subsystems could be to dissociate thinking from feeling and movement, or feeling from movement and action, etc. Three different forms of armouring are therefore recognised: visceral, with disturbances of gut and ventilation; muscular, with disturbances of tone and fluid dynamics (and therefore cardiovascular disease); and cerebral, with disturbances of perception and insight.

Boadella refers to a person's 'inner ground' by which he means the essential qualities or essence of a person ('soul' would appear to be a perfectly good synonym). The inner ground should ideally be perfectly embodied in the soma, which, in turn, would be perfectly energised. Biosynthesis is therefore transphysical, vitalistic and descriptively somatic.

Therapeutic work in biosynthesis is related to the integration of dysfunction as perceived according to the model. It involves working directly with breathing and its emotional associations; grounding and its association with movement and expressive energy patterns through the body; 'facing and sounding' which refers to working with the eyes, voice and language; and attention to the inner ground, or spiritual awareness. Touch is used to communicate a variety of experiences to the patient, such as the solidity of self or of another human being, the flow of energy, the rhythm of involuntary body motion, or warmth.

Boadella writes:

> 'A person's uniqueness is grounded in the physical body, and embodied in the tissues. So the qualities of personal life are reflected in qualities of muscle tone, facial expression, breathing rhythms and organisation of excitement. The practitioner sees people whose bodies have been conditioned by the restrictive images they took on from their internalisation of environmental demands. To see a person clearly is to see through these restrictive images encapsulated in the character, and beyond the constricted conditions imposed by the muscular armour.' (Rowan & Dryden 1990, p 157)

Biodynamic therapy

This system is considered here in a little detail because it is centred upon working with the body probably to a greater extent than in bioenergetics (which it closely resembles) or biosynthesis. Like biosynthesis, it is based upon a vitalistic concept of life force, which, in addition to its more animal excitatory and pleasure-giving nature, is described as capable of facilitating the 'ethical personality' — the developed individual. This is said to occur because the vital energy may resonate at a lofty height with universal values — a somewhat Platonic notion. Practitioners therefore, encourage free association, regression and catharsis, confident that there will be balance between emotional expression and adequate control. Such confidence is based upon the practitioner's ability to encourage either the 'upward' or the 'downward' phase of emotional cycles described below. The life force, also described as the libido, is perceived in this model as a physiological, psychological and cosmological reality. Used in this way, the device of the libido therefore conveniently straddles — or dispenses with — more than the usual philosophical difficulties.

Gerda Boyesen, the originator of biodynamic therapy, trained in physiotherapy after (Freudian) psychology, so convinced was she that it was necessary to work with the body as an adjunct to verbal psychotherapy. She began by combining psychotherapy with massage and collecting observations of the relationship between somatic and simultaneous psychological events. She was particularly interested in:

- the changing quality of bowel sounds (stethoscopically observed) with emotional processing, and
- the build up and release of bodily tissue fluid, correlating with emotional build up and discharge.

One central emphasis is that, within a person, there are unresolved cycles of emotional charge and discharge (see also the work of Stanley Keleman, above). The cycles are also bodily or physiological events, described as the emotional vasomotor cycle. For example, the life force or libido, which is seen as originating in the viscera, may, during an interpersonal transaction, be built up as a feeling of anger (with associated angry thoughts). But it is also embodied as increasing expressive muscular tension. With appropriate discharge of emotional energy, relaxation of muscles and 'psychoperistalsis', the reconciliatory, reorganisational calming of the person can properly occur without interruption. Psychoperistalsis is the name given to a process whereby the gut literally digests the vegetative after-effects of emotional stress. The calm termination of the cycle in which psychoperistalsis takes part is crucial after such a psychophysiological disruption.

The libido is seen as originating at a vegetative core level. It intrinsically always tends to express itself fully, streaming through to the surface of the body. Ideally, this movement of energy should involve appropriate and temporary patterns of muscular tone, fluid movement, breathing dynamics and vocal expression in an integrative, cyclical wave. 'The life force moves in us as libido, its flow being intrinsically pleasurable except if it is blocked, when it causes symptoms both physical and psychological.' (Southwell 1990, p 180). In essence, the task of the practitioner is to facilitate the unblocking of this integrated flow through the three levels of viscera, muscle and psyche. The three levels correspond with the three embryological layers in biosynthesis.

Important to this analysis is the concept of the *horizontal* muscular (ego) regulation and expression of the *vertical* upsurge of raw (id) emotion (a Reichian idea). The vertical wave of emotion may be over-controlled or inadequately controlled at a muscular level, but also at a visceral and psychological level, as a result of inadequacies in the child's nurturing environment. If, for example, the life force is interrupted from completing its movement through the three levels, then it accumulates in the body tissue as unresolved pressures capable of causing psychological or somatic disorder. In this case the person may remain partly locked in an unresolved emotional experience by, for example, retaining a residue of guilt from the non-acceptance of felt anger. This might involve remaining rigid at a muscular level, and unable to let go of muscular tensions which are the normal accompaniment to emotional events. At the deeply vegetative visceral level, it might involve retaining a residue of fluid pressure and other undigested, physiologically represented, emotional stress.

Overcontrolled persons, unaware of the possible richness of their own emotional and physical life, are caricatured typically as winning social approval. They achieve this by repressing the heart and gut feelings, by being too reasonable and keeping the stiff upper lip. This kind of caricature and summary is not, of course, exclusive to biodynamic therapy. Although body armouring is a concept accepted and respected by most schools of psychology, the explicitly visceral level of expression and assimilation of experience, together with the cyclical concept of energy flow, is perhaps the trademark of biodynamics.

Biodynamic techniques

Quite apart from the character of verbal, psychotherapeutic interactions in biodynamic therapy which need not concern us here, touching and bodywork is a major tool. Massage is used extensively to melt or soften the body armour, and may typically involve weekly treatment for several months. This use of massage involves a greater regularity and prolongation of treatment than its more common use for simple relaxation or periodic stress relief. As discussed briefly above, the aetiology of muscle tension is seen as exclusively psychological and, furthermore, it is seen as being intimately connected with suppressed patterns of ventilation. Biodynamic therapists try to encourage and facilitate the appropriate bodily resurgence of emotional events which have been historically interrupted at the upward phase of the cycle. They may also encourage the calming of muscular energy through its distribution in the downward phase of the cycle.

The practitioner uses the stethoscope in order to interpret the language of bowel sounds in response to the emotional processing:

> '*Dry, percussive sounds tell us we are softening some fibres in the chronic muscle armour; sounds like thunder tell us we are moving excess fluid out of the tissue; gentle continuous sounds like a babbling brook tell us that the life force is flowing harmoniously. The more watery the sounds the riper is the life force that we are mobilizing; the drier the sounds the more deeply the dynamic is buried.*' (Rowan & Dryden 1988, p 193)

Massage is used to deepen the patient's sense of inner presence and self-awareness. As a result, the patient makes contact with, and is able to respond to those inner stirrings which are the inexorable streamings of libidinous life force. Massage is therefore perceived as a vitally important form of communication within the whole person's fullness of depth.

Biodynamic vegetotherapy is a term given to the process of encouraging free association with thoughts, feelings, bodily sensations and movements. It is a kind of authentic movement on a biological and emotional level, whereby spontaneous bodily movements or inner sensations are watched for by practitioner and client. When detected, they are encouraged to expand and be fully felt; allowed to grow into the fullness of expression. This attention to inner promptings is a commonly used psychotherapeutic technique.

As a précis, the attention of biodynamic work is upon unresolved cycles of emotional and physiological bodily charge and discharge, strongly locating the person within his or her body.

Bioenergetics, biosynthesis and biodynamic therapy are representative of a fast-growing population of psychologically trained practitioners who are choosing to work with the body, and providing variations on a similar model of psychosomatic integration. Traditionally, the mind and the body have received forms of attention characterised by separate disciplines and even separate styles of language. Latterly, it has become more fashionable to speak of the body-mind and of mind/body integration. But to encourage the synthesis, it is tempting to replace these clumsy terms with 'self', and to explore the consequences. Kepner, a gestalt psychotherapist, has provided a detailed exploration of the effect of this exercise, and his work is the most readily accessible and insightful treatise on body/mind integration. The following section draws heavily upon Kepner's description of gestalt body-work in *Body Process: Working with the Body in Psychotherapy* (Kepner 1993).

GESTALT THERAPY AND THE SELF

The founder of gestalt therapy, Frederick Perls, was himself a client of Reich and was intensely interested in Reich's theories of somatic psychotherapy. Like Reichian therapy, gestalt therapy is therefore very biological and primarily centres upon the bodily experience of the self; dealing with the withholding of expression is the secondary consideration. Because gestalt theory is concerned with the experience of sensations of the embodied self, it lends itself both to the current interest in phenomenology in medical thought, and to the incorporation process currently afoot in the psychological sciences.

The task in gestalt therapy is the gradual development of full awareness and ownership of one's bodily existence. Kepner argues (as Perls did) that the term 'armour' (as in body armour) is a negative one, because muscular constrictions represent the patient's creative approach to integrating physical and emotional insult into the self. Therefore, working with the body should not be intrusive and militaristic, as in Reich's 'breaking down resistance to proper functioning'. Instead, it should involve the re-sensing and re-owning of those parts of the self that were used to maintain function in the presence of insult.[7] For gestalt therapists, the emotional meanings of posture and tension are just as important as the expression they prevent. Rather than be defeated, these resistances must be reintegrated into the self to allow a wholer functioning.

Kepner describes in some detail the process of decorporation of human beings which has taken place in Western societies, especially with respect to disowned parts of the self. He points out that when we say 'I', we are referring to a self which seems independent of the body, whereas when we say 'my body', it is as if the body is a possession, like a car. This shows that there is thus an I–it relationship involved with reference to one's body, whereas there is no one word that explicitly includes the body, when referring to the self. Our language supports the notion that bodies are objects; that my body is something that happens to me, rather than the me that is happening (Kepner 1993, p 7). Being removed from bodily experience means that things seem to happen to us — hence we feel out of control or fragmented or desensitised. We may not feel ourselves.

The body as 'it' has the effect of rendering ourselves less than we really are, because we cut off a part of ourselves from our awareness. If I am struggling to solve the problems of relationships and live a meaningful life, then since 'I' does not include my body, the body is seen as irrelevant to these struggles. But nothing could be further from the truth.

> *'We live not only through our thinking and imagining, but also through moving, posturing, sensing, expressing. How, then, can we ignore the fundamental physical nature of the person in a profession [psychotherapy] where the aim is to heal the self, the whole person?'* (Kepner 1993, p 1)

Hence the concept of the embodied self is central to the gestalt view. In so far as this view argues effectively for the integration of the body into the concept of the self, which has hitherto been regarded as 'elusive and ephemeral' (Kepner 1993, p 10), it is of great use to manual practitioners. But it should be pointed out that the gestalt view sees the self *only* as a process, attributing to it no intrinsic nature of its own. The gestalt body-self allows for a sophisticated treatise on the nature of excitation and withdrawal — and here is its great strength — but some may find its reduction of the human condition to one of mere transactional functioning restrictive. It is, of course, poor biological functioning which is so palpable to manual practitioners, and so since the gestalt view has much to say on this subject, it is worthy of serious study.

The crucial fact for manual practitioners and gestalt body-process practitioners is that the body is actually the locus or site of the disowned self; the body-self *is* the disowned part of the self. Why is this so? Because the functions it seems necessary to disown are either explicitly physical or rooted in the physical nature. It is possible simultaneously physically to deaden sensations of love, anger and so on, by tensing against them, and prevent the muscular movements associated with them. This suppressive and masking effect of muscles has been described in previous sections. It is precisely because affect and emotion are body phenomena that the disowning of emotional life involves the disowning of the body-self. Similarly, it is precisely because emotion is matured and unfolded in expressive muscular movement that the body-self is disowned when emotional expression as movement is suppressed. And because movement is what gives meaning to emotion, that is, it allows need to make contact with environment, then meaning, understandability and the significance of emotions are disowned along with the body. Pain and sexuality are disowned for the same reasons. (Kepner 1993, ch. 2)

Furthermore, because body language is not a verbal one, but, as we have seen, a kinaesthetic, symbolic, irrational, emotional one, then the body-self seems nonsensical and cannot adequately be verbalised. On the other hand, the 'I', the apparent self, is readily identified with emotionless thought and intellectual processes.

Of the many techniques gestalt therapists may use to encourage reownership of bodily experience, Kepner describes a simple exercise in body self-awareness (Kepner 1993, p 8), beginning with the attributing of perceived tension in the shoulders to a process of the self. For example, the statement 'I feel tension in the shoulders' becomes 'I am tensing my shoulders'. Many people resist the notion that they are tensing their shoulders even though it is clear that no one else is doing it. They do this because they persist in using the I–it attitude towards their bodies. Tension is a self-organised act in response to a stimulus. My act of tensing my shoulders may not be sufficiently experienced by and *as* myself in order for me to realise that it is me who is doing it.

The experiment continues to merge subject and object; 'I am tensing my self, I am tense in my shoulders' and so on. Further descriptions of the sensation are encouraged — eg compressing, containing, etc, but with the verbal structure 'I am containing myself, and this is my existence'. The idea is to feel the impact of considering one's bodily state to be descriptive of one's existential state, which encourages reownership of split-off parts of the self. In instances where the experiment seems not to get anywhere, this too is given bodily and existential expression: 'I don't feel comfortable attending to my body, and this is my existence', or 'my body is trivial, and this is my experience', 'I don't feel much of myself and this is my experience', and so on.

But the bulk of gestalt theory is concerned with the cycle of experience, a process that involves becoming aware of needs, mobilising the body in order to contact the environment so as to find completion for needs, experiencing satisfaction and finally withdrawing. Unlike the other cycles described in this chapter, it is not based upon the fight/flight reaction but is much more general and considerably more sophisticated. Whilst it is not appropriate to review this concept here, its importance for practitioners of manual medicine lies in the elaborate description of types of bodily 'disownership' that can occur, according to how and at what stage the cycle of experience is interrupted. Interruption therefore involves the interference with sensations and movements, where an intricate and detailed continuum exists from the former to the latter, and back to the (new) former again.

A FREUDIAN EXPLANATION FOR OSTEOPATHIC TREATMENT

Randell (1992, unpublished lecture 1997) proposes a Freudian osteopathic clinical rationale, which has already been mentioned earlier in this chapter, but deserves more attention at its conclusion. Randell argues that, far from being physicians who are best at helping with 'surgically unstable spinal disease' (a premise not substantiated), osteopaths [and other manipulators] are in reality hypnotists, whose field of influence is over psychically determined disorders. In saying this, Randell is making at least two familiar assertions: one, that the cause of problems manipulative therapists deal with is largely psychological; and two, that the mechanical rationale underlying osteopathy is naïve and false.

Randell argues that 'biopathic bodily fixations and rigidities [ie those diagnostic findings apprehended by osteopaths] represent somatised defences against primitive anxieties'. These are created when 'the force of the child's libidinal excitement encounters either emphatic non-acceptance or alternatively perversely precocious stimulation by the parent or surrogate'.

Some of the child's natural urges for self-expression, assertion and preservation, involving expansive movement patterns, glandular stimulation and their accompanying sensations, are forbidden or overstimulated. The resultant blocking or repression of normal expression is a trauma represented by 'involuntary muscular tension and rigidity which bind [silence] these sensations and thus protect against mental pain and suffering'.

Since these processes are initiated at a preverbal level, this aspect of somatic character structure is a learned, conditioned, sensation continuum and a motor taboo. That is, certain types of arousal and urges to motility are inhibited for fear of releasing traumatic impulses and sensations. To begin with, the taboos represent movements which the infant *will* not do, and sensations which the infant *will* not allow itself, for fear of parental disapproval. But as the child develops, the 'will not' becomes a 'can not' because it is selected out of the range of possibilities of movement and feelings. It is then locked out with appropriate patterns of myofascial rigidity and other tissue equivalents.

For Randell's theory of what occurs in treatment, it is important that much if not all of the entire somatic dimension of character structure (which osteopathy and similar therapeutics are apparently suited to address) represent the internalised will or ego of the parent. The parental will therefore contaminates the patient's conscience and its influence over bodily life, structure and function.

Transference and the patient/practitioner relationship ✂

The special inhibitions and suppressions, that is, the alterations of the child's and later the adult's normal expressive life, because they were once forced by the parents, therefore require similar submission to authority in order to be resolved. So it is a condition, in this interpretation of the encounter, that the practitioner is associated in the patient's unconscious with the image of a parent figure. Likewise, the patient is, in Randell's words, 'caught as a child'. The theory depends upon this formation, in the therapeutic encounter, of a parent/child relationship, rather than an adult/adult one.

This transference process is assisted by many of the usual features of the consultation — especially power-discrepancy. Power-discrepancy exists in the context of: the patient's disrobing, being prostrate, being moved and acted upon by one with mysterious knowledge, higher status, perhaps social standing, etc. The diminished power and will of the patient may therefore succumb more easily to the influence of a new, more powerful practitioner's will. The patient is always encouraged to relax as much as possible during treatment (except during occasional procedures which require the patient's muscular participation). This reduces the presence of the *motor* body-self ('The ego is first and foremost a body ego', (Freud 1927)). Since the ego finds final outward expression in movement, then if the will to movement is diminished, then its role in the whole interaction is considerably lessened and restricted to verbal interaction (which may well be minimal).

The infantile need for physical contact persists into adulthood and is likely to become more intense in periods of stress and loss where those much earlier feelings of peril are reawakened. The tendency of the self to regress to a helpless, child-like state when being handled and passive, and when being in the sick role, no doubt assists the creation in the patient's mind of the parent/adult type of relationship and a hypnotic state. When the movements being applied are rhythmic and repetitive, this hypnotic effect is likely to be increased as resonance occurs with body-memory of infant rocking by the mother (see Ch. 3). Movements applied by the practitioner's 'more capable hands' to the patient's body with the patient in this hypnotised, childlike state, are far from being mechanical fix-its. Instead they are new, preverbal, motor suggestions and sensations, which can unfasten the previous autosuggestive inhibitions and free the patient from her self-induced spell.

Randell further injects Freudian sexology into the theory by caricaturing the two polar types of treatment. 'Father' hypnosis involves powerful suggestion, where the manipulations are more sudden and firm, accompanied perhaps by feelings of fear, shock and cathartic phenomena; for example, high velocity thrust techniques. 'Mother' hypnosis involves seductive suggestion, where the techniques are gentle, slow and involve holding, containing; for example, functional or so-called craniosacral techniques. Because these movements are done or encouraged or forced by parental authority figures, they are once again permitted by the body-self. Hence a manipulative practitioner is always a type of surrogate parent to the patient.

This species of theory will by now be familiar to the reader. What is especially important for any emerging psychosomatic theory of manipulative therapy is the question of the nature of the patient/ practitioner relationship. Latey (1997a, personal communication 1997) opposes the view that the parent/adult resonance is in any way desirable. His view is that if it does occur it tends to cause habitual unrealistic and unhelpful properties in the therapeutic relationship which can prevent proper resolution of long-term psychosomatic problems. Latey insists that practitioners should take great care to manoeuvre away from being seen as parental figures, lover figures, authority figures, or child figures, in order to avoid limitation of progress (Latey 1997a,c). Latey's view is an important one, being probably representative of the most progressive psychosomatic thinking in manual therapy. But it is vital to reconcile his antitransference view with the argument in favour of the use of infantile body-memory triggered by manual therapy.

A need for psychological science in manual therapy?

By relinquishing ego control of body movements into 'more capable hands', the patient renders that part of her unconscious which organises bodily movements and sensations directly in contact with the practitioner. Movements and sensations occurring in the patient's body as a result of the physician's ministrations will therefore be significant at a distinctly unconscious level. They may be framed by early parental relationships. Randell claims not only that transference occurs in any case in manual therapy (by no means a new notion), but that it should be utilised, and that it explains how manipulative therapy works. If this is correct, or desirable, then manual practitioners must:

- learn basic depth psychology
- subject themselves to a minimum of self-reflection, to be able to work with or around transference and carry the treatment forward.

In these circumstances, the necessity for supervision in manual medicine would become central.

Randell argues that a knowledge of the theory and use of depth psychology is necessary to transform the practice of manual therapy from a partitive pseudoscience into a respectable discipline; one that is capable of offering relief for the 'epidemic of psychogenic, somatising disorders which threaten to engulf orthodox medical services' (Randell 1992).

The theory asserts, then, that the practitioners of manual and manipulative therapy have considerably more contact with and influence over unconscious aspects of the patient's psyche than is normally thought. The implication of the theory is that the psyche, as much as the body, is that which is capable of being manipulated during manual therapy. The notion of a manual practitioner working explicitly as a parent archetype is a highly controversial one. In today's ethically aware patient population with its quest for autonomy, informed consent and non-paternalistic intervention, the psychological power-play and the potential for its abuse may be cause for concern. There already exist strong objections to the use of power and transference within the psychotherapeutic profession (Masson 1990, 1992).

Randell argues that the fixations of body armouring predispose to many subsequent structural pathologies in both musculoskeletal and visceral tissues. For anywhere where irritable neuromotor tissue is found, sensitive manipulative therapy is therefore the treatment of choice. He maintains that this theory paves the ways to the understanding of dysfunction of cardiovascular, respiratory and gastrointestinal systems as well as those of the musculoskeletal system (all of which are notoriously lacking in sound aetiological theories in orthodox texts). In this respect he is no different from the other psychosomaticists described in the chapter. None, however, gives the theory such a classically Freudian context, and none has worked so hard to give the arguments concerning aetiology a biological basis.

Randell's version ignores the possibility that traumatic mechanical forces from outside, with or without the help of other environmental phenomena, could be responsible for myofascial hypertonia. He assumes causative factors are primarily psychological or otherwise relatively unimportant. This is reminiscent of the fact that physiologico-mechanical theorists have likewise ignored the psycho-dynamic possibilities.

SUMMARY OF MAIN POINTS

This chapter has:

1. shown that the use of touch and the refusal to use it, in psychotherapy, exposes its extreme psychological significance. This opens the way, yet again, for the possibility of an emergent psychological understanding of the dynamics of manual therapy.

2. challenged the notion that muscular hypertonia is usually caused by anything other than centrally ordered, psychological processes (except in the case of obvious tissue damage).

3. explored certain psychological attitudes towards the body and its formation. These strongly suggest that emotional phenomena are causative with respect to structure and function of the body-self. It has touched on the notion of body form as having meaning.

4. looked briefly at some models which attempt to integrate mind and body in the realms of psychotherapeutic bodywork and manual medicine.

CONCLUSIONS

Psychotherapists working with the body are dealing with painful sensations and muscular tensions of the kinds with which manual therapists also regularly deal. This premise is unresearched. However, it is unreasonable to assume that the patient populations of these two disciplines differ markedly in their basic constitutional make-up — especially with respect to the aetiology of muscular hypertonia. It is simply likely that patients are selecting those practitioners from whom they imagine themselves deriving benefit. They will have special reasons for doing this, probably according to inherent qualities of self-awareness.

Bodyworking psychotherapists assert that, only by being made aware of cut-off parts of the self, which are largely located in the body, might patients realise that it is they who are creating the tensions and awkward feelings, and not some strange and dissociated outer force ('the leg is stiff'). Therefore the focus of their work is to bring back into the patient's awareness the body as self. It demands the full cognitive participation of the patient in both verbalised and body-oriented aspects of therapy. One of the strengths of proposals of these sorts is in an improved understanding of patterns of muscular rigidity for which there is no other reasonable explanation.

This point immediately finds an echo in Lederman's work (mentioned in Chapter 2). His research suggests that, where motor functions are to be treated, and not merely certain tissue properties (structural tissue damage due to mechanical stress and overuse), then the patient must take an active role in rehabilitation and manual therapy. This is because the motor system is not amenable to alteration by purely passive manipulation. In particular, 'reflexive-type treatment aiming to stimulate the lower motor system is ineffective' (Lederman 1997, p 145). According to Lederman, central, cognitive control is over-riding and needs to be involved in manual therapy for best results. This means that only by the direct involvement of the psyche is it possible to initiate those plastic changes in neuromuscular tone which can bring about gross changes in body textures and postures. 'Possibly the only treatment to have any longlasting effect is one which communicates with the patient and encourages movement which is cognitive and volitional.' (Lederman 1997, p 145) This is very similar to the gestalt view.

If gestalt theory and Lederman's theory are sufficient explanations, then standard manual therapy as it is widely practised cannot bring about the improvements in postural, muscular and visceral problems which are claimed to occur. It would be argued that it is unable to produce the changes in motor tone which would be necessary for such healing to occur. Instead, manipulative therapy can only be operating in the realms of mechanical stress and overuse in muscle tissue, because any modulation of the motor system has to involve the patient's cognition, volition, and preferably active movements. But most manual practitioners do not work in this way.

Manipulative and other manual therapy involving techniques performed upon a passive patient are the norm and have been efficacious for over a century. If reports of regular and considerable changes in muscle motor tone and the defacilitation of hyper-irritable spinal reflexes due to passive treatment are to be believed (which they ought to be, considering the palpatory skill of practitioners), then something else must be happening besides the purely mechanical effects of manipulation on tissue. Instead, if the *self* must be involved in the reclaiming of neurologically dissociated bodily functions, then manual therapy functions also with the higher centres of the unconscious self. But it need not involve the explicitly conscious job of integrating previously disowned parts of the self. Motor changes *may* happen spontaneously because the cognitive–emotional self is involved, but at a vegetative and preconscious level.

What this means is that the ability of manual therapy to activate unconscious psychological events has been grossly underestimated — by the manual medicine professions. It is likely that these events are responsible for the beneficial changes in the motor system previously attributed to simple relexogenic mechanisms.

This important conclusion would concur with Latey's insistence that psychotherapeutic techniques are not necessary in manual therapy, even when dealing with long-term psychosomatic problems (Latey 1997b,c). This is because integration and healing happens at an unconscious level, as a result of the special mixture of bodywork together with simple, thoughtful and mature adult-to-adult conversation involving use of humour and metaphor (Latey 1997b,c,d). He maintains the process is hindered by transference and regression, and that these phenomena can be dispensed with. However, Latey himself cites his references in the realms of depth psychology and psychoanalysis, and it is not at all clear from his writings whether or not his techniques are partly verbal interventions of a sort which psychotherapists would recognise as being typical of their work.

The conclusion would also concur with Randell's description of manipulative therapy as a form of hypnotherapy, but which, conversely, has its *basis* in transference and regression. One of the important open questions left hanging at the outset of manual therapy — as psychologically influential, therefore, — is that concerning the nature of the patient/practitioner relationship, and how it should be cultivated.

The notion of psychologically significant manual therapy would furthermore concur with a theory of the self which is truly integrated.

Psychotherapists and psychoanalysts have always maintained that the self can heal through psychotherapeutic conversation in its various forms, without explicit reference to, or working upon, the body. If the self is a unitary body-self then there is no reason why the converse should not also be true — namely, that sensitive bodywork, without the use of explicit psychotherapeutic techniques, can also facilitate healing of that same self. If mental and physical self are a unity, then together they are available to both psychological and somatic forms of therapy. That this should be so rests on the notion that healing can be triggered by the slightest stimulus, if that stimulus is well placed.[8]

Research into structure and function of the brain strongly suggests that all visceral, humoral and other autonomic functions, in addition to those involving movement and sensation, achieve a highly charged, cortical representation. The mind in brain form, therefore, is aware of, and cannot be excluded from any explanation of disease processes because the neocortex can detect, register and categorise somatic events which constantly flood into it via afferent systems. According to the Frankl–Randell theory of psychosomatic biopathy (Randell, unpublished lecture, 1997), the presence of this continuum of sensation, presented to the mind, is the necessary condition for the discharge and expression of appropriate responses to it. (These instinctual urges are coded for in the cingulate cortex on the medial face of the frontal lobe.) In cases where the individual has suffered repeated psychological trauma, these representation of bodily perceptions are chronically inhibited and the responses to them paralysed. As a sort of compensation for this damming of neural energy, a state of chronic hyper-arousal develops in the anterior cingulate area, resulting in a chronic but incoherent efferent discharge into the soma. That is, the prefrontal system projects incongruently on to the body, via the output pyramids of the anterior cingulate area, neural events which it fears would be rejected if congruently expressed. This inappropriate and disoriented neural output into effector systems not only explains chronic muscular hypertonia, but also provides a baseline explanation for all psychosomatic pathology.

If this is a correct explanation of fundamental events, then the underlying theory behind all explanations of psychosomatics alluded to in this chapter — that traumatic suppression of emotional life results in bodily dysfunction — is gradually being validated by advances in the understanding of neural functioning and brain imaging techniques. As such technology improves, the psycho-neurological implications will need to be absorbed by the somatic therapies in order to avoid embarrassing gaps in theory. Manual medicine rationale would therefore do well to consider redefin-ing its concepts and methods. If it is possible to change psycho-logical characteristics through bodywork, then this is evidence of the myth of body/mind duality, or at least of the notion that body/mind separation is largely for culturally derived concepts of being. If the authors referenced in this chapter are correct in attributing psychological life to flesh, then should not manual therapists add some of these working hypotheses to their clinical rationales?

Each person speaks through her body of those attitudes and feelings which she finds easy and natural to express from minute to minute, and which are understood by anyone (from the same culture). But each speaks just as eloquently of those past traumata, shocks and assaults on her being which have resulted in patterns of rigidity, constriction, inhibited movements, neuronal interruptions, stagnations, and so on. These somatic codes may be interpretable only by those who have developed the necessary observational skills. Manual practitioners, with their extraordinarily fine palpatory abilities, have more to offer and explore than they could currently possibly imagine in the realm of human distress. It is merely necessary for them to cease to pretend that the human body is a mechanical device, and instead absorb and utilise psychological con-cepts which integrate the body into the self.

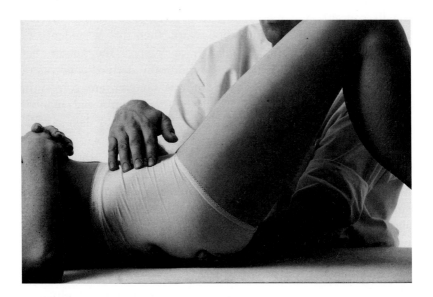

NOTES

[1]For discussions of the problems inherent in psychotherapy and physical contact with respect to sexuality and aggression, see Masson (1990), Rutter (1991) and Jehu (1994).

[2]For example, osteopathy, chiropractic, manipulative physiotherapy, craniosacral therapy, kinesiology, Rolfing, shiatsu, aromatherapy, reflexology, body-harmony, reiki, therapeutic massage – sports, remedial and others – polarity therapy and other species of manual healing, not to mention non-manual but body-oriented health-focused activities such as Tai Chi, Chi Kung, dance therapy, Feldenkreis, Alexander and other body arts.

[3]In body psychology theory it is not merely abnormal muscular components that are considered to have psychological cause. Visceral dysfunction is ascribed to the same mechanisms. See bioenergetics, biosynthesis and biodynamic therapy.

[4]Although this author allows for the conversion of stress-induced motor tone to structural muscle tone in his classification of abnormal tone, he does not describe it specifically.

[5]James Kepner's *Body Process: Working with the Body in Psychotherapy* (1993) is perhaps the most outstanding work in this field. It is not only the younger or fringe psychotherapeutic disciplines that are moving in the direction of the body; the Jungian and psychoanalytic schools, traditionally rooted in the symbolic and intellectual, are also recognising the intrinsic involvement of bodily being in human process (Kepner 1993, p xvi).

[6]Analogously, osteopaths have noted that despite the spinal column's obvious segmental arrangement, this is merely to allow the need for movement and the emergence of spinal nerves to coexist. The neural tissue in the spinal cord is not organised into horizontal bands, but into sets of non-layered vertical motor patterns corresponding with movements involving the coordination of muscles and other tissues throughout the length and breadth of the body.

[7]Don McFarland (McFarland 1988), a seasoned bodyworker and formulator of the technique of 'body harmony', argues that manual practitioners should *never* inflict pain. Rather, practitioners should work to facilitate and allow tensions to unwind without the kind of confrontation which tends to increase resistance.

[8]David Taylor Reilly's concept and practice of the 'therapeutic consultation' likewise relies upon huge, whole-person shifts of a profoundly healing nature with very little apparent physician activity (Reilly 1996).

REFERENCES

Baron R J 1992 Why aren't more physicians phenomenologists? In: Leder D (ed) The body in medical thought and practice. Philosophy and Medicine Series vol. 43, Kluwer Academic Publishers, Dordrecht, p 17–36
Boadella D 1987 Lifestreams: an introduction to biosynthesis. Routledge, London
Boadella D 1990 Biosynthesis. In: Rowan J, Dryden W (eds) Innovative therapy in Britain. Open University Press, Buckingham
Boyesen G 1982 The primary personality. Journal of Biodynamic Psychology 3: 3–8
Boyesen G 1985 Entre psyche et soma. Payot, Paris
Bradford S 1965 Role of osteopathic manipulative therapy in emotional disorders: a physiologic hypothesis. Journal of the American Medical Association 64: 484–493
Chaitow L 1997 Palpation skills: assessment and diagnosis through touch. Churchill Livingstone, Edinburgh

Dunn F 1948 The osteopathic management of psychosomatic problems. Journal of the American Osteopathic Association 48(4): 196–199

Freud S 1927 The ego and the id. Trans. J Riviere. Hogarth, London

Hoffman S, Gazit M 1996 To touch and be touched in psychotherapy. Changes: An International Journal of Psychology and Psychotherapy 14(2): 115–116

Hope Robertson R c.1938 Booklet outlining a proposal for a British osteopathic mental hospital. In: Collins M 1994 Views of the past. British Osteopathic Journal 13: 42–43

Jehu D 1994 Patients as victims: sexual abuse in psychotherapy and counselling. John Wiley, Chichester

Keleman S 1985 Emotional anatomy. Center Press, Berkeley

Kepner J I 1993 Body process: working with the body in psychotherapy. Jossey-Bass, San Francisco

Kertay L, Reviere S L 1993 The use of touch in psychotherapy: theoretical and ethical considerations. Psychotherapy 30(1): 32–40

Kurtz R, Prestera H 1984 The body reveals. Harper and Row, New York

Latey P 1982 The muscular manifesto. Self-published, UK

Latey P 1996 Feelings, muscles and movement. Journal of Bodywork and Movement Therapies 1(1): 44–52

Latey P 1997a Maturation – the evolution of psychosomatic problems: migraine and asthma. Journal of Bodywork and Movement Therapies 1(2): 107–116

Latey P 1997b Basic clinical tactics. Journal of Bodywork and Movement Therapies 1(3): 163–172

Latey P 1997c The balance of practice: preparing for long-term work. Journal of Bodywork and Movement Therapies 1(4): 223–230

Latey P 1997d Complexity and the changing individual. Journal of Bodywork and Movement Therapies 1(5): 270–279

Leder D 1990 The absent body, University of Chicago Press, Chicago

Lederman E 1997 Fundamentals of manual therapy. Churchill Livingstone, Edinburgh

Lowen A 1976 The language of the body. Macmillan, New York

Lowen A 1994 Bioenergetics. Arkana, New York

McFarland D 1988 Body secrets. Healing Arts Press, Los Angeles

Masson J 1990 Against therapy. Fontana, London

Masson J 1992 Final analysis. Fontana, London

Painter J 1987 Deep bodywork and personal development. Bodymind Books, California

Perls F S, Hefferline R F, Goodman P 1951 Gestalt therapy. Julian, New York

Randell P 1992 The crisis of clinical theory supporting osteopathic practice: a critique and new proposal. British Osteopathic Journal 9: 5–7

Reich W 1933, 1991 Character analysis. Noonday Press, New York

Reilly D 1996 Creating therapeutic consultations. Audiotape of lecture given at conference, The Placebo Response: Biology and Belief, University of Westminster, London (Tapes available from the Scientific and Medical Network, UK)

Rowan J, Dryden W (eds) 1990 Innovative therapy in Britain. Open University Press, Buckingham

Rutter P 1991 Sex in the forbidden zone. Mandala, London

Sayers J 1996 On kissing, touching and shaking hands. Changes: An International Journal of Psychology and Psychotherapy 14(2): 117–120

Schwartz H S (ed) 1973 Mental health and chiropractic – a multidisciplinary approach. Sessions, New York

Shaw R 1996 Towards integrating the body in psychotherapy. Changes: An International Journal of Psychology and Psychotherapy 14(2): 108–114

Sheldrake R 1985 A new science of life: the hypothesis of formative causation. Anthony Blond, London

Southwell C 1990 The Gerda Boyesen method: biodynamic therapy. In: Rowan J, Dryden W (eds) Innovative therapy in Britain. Open University Press, Buckingham
Still A T 1908 Autobiography. Published by the author, Kirksville, MO. Reprinted in 1981 by the American Academy of Osteopathy
Whitfield G 1990 Bioenergetics. In: Rowan J, Dryden W (eds) Innovative therapy in Britain. Open University Press, Buckingham
Wilson J 1982 The value of touch in psychotherapy. American Journal of Orthopsychiatry 52(1): 65–72
Woodmansey A C 1988 Are psychotherapists out of touch? British Journal of Psychotherapy 5(1): 57–65

PSYCHOLOGY FURTHER READING: biodynamic therapy, biosynthesis and bioenergetics

Boadella D 1985 Wilhelm Reich: the evolution of his work. Routledge & Kegan Paul, London
Boyesen M-L 1974 Psycho-peristalsis 1: the abdominal discharge of nervous tension. Energy and Character 5(1): 5–16
Boyesen M-L 1975 Psycho-peristalsis V: function of the libido circulation. Energy and Character 6(3): 61–68
The Collected Papers of Biodynamic Psychology, vols 1, 2 1980. Biodynamic Publications, London
Journal of Biodynamic Psychology Nos 1, 2, 3. Biodynamic Publications, London
Lowen A 1969 The betrayal of the body. Macmillan, London
Millenson J 1995 Mind matters: psychological medicine in holistic practice, Eastland Press, Seattle
Smith E 1985 The body in psychotherapy. McFarland, Jefferson
Southwell C 1982 Biodynamic massage as a therapeutic tool. Journal of Biodynamic Psychology 3: 40–54

5

Conclusions

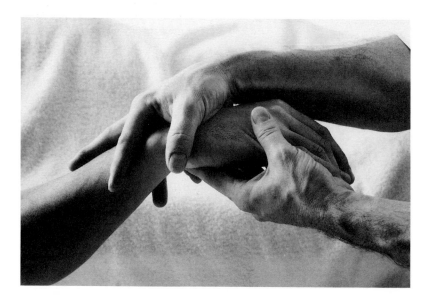

PHENOMENOLOGY

The phenomenological perspective

Phenomenology involves using the language of experience to form the ground of philosophical investigation, and therefore to form the basis of discussions of the human condition. Phenomenology is important because it avoids the use of those terms of reference that separate mind and body. It proceeds instead by using a different language structure; speaking of flesh as lived, self or mind as embodied. The essentially corporeal, subjective experience of each person is considered as the ground for descriptions of the world. This has the effect of dissolving away the idea that the mind is another 'substance' alongside the body. Phenomenology is becoming the philosophical mode of choice in medical theory and ecology and as such deserves mention at the conclusion of this text.

The basic phenomenological view of the body is that it can never be just another object in the world, because it is *that which brings the world about.* The body is both the subject and object; it both discloses the world and is part that world. Fleshly being is therefore a special kind, incapable of being wholly objectified. The 'lived body' is where human thought, feeling, decision, experience, activity is lived out and such life is imprinted, sedimented, embodied through each fibre of tissue (Leder 1992).

For example, although my perceptive apparatus may be available in a certain sense to the experience of a scientist, it can never be available to me, because it is absorbed into my 'means whereby things become available' (Leder 1990, Ch. 1). Crucially, though, it is never available to the scientist as the means of perception. The sense organs, therefore, can never be a thing, like other inanimate things in the world. This argument holds true for the whole of the body.

The body is the means whereby we perceive the world, and act in it, and yet it is clearly (at least partly) *of* the world. It is thereby a mysterious duality in itself, not merely flesh but ensouled flesh. We may experience our bodies, but only from within themselves as the agents of the experience. This view of the body is integrative. It demands an undeviating attention to the body as the primary context for experience and activity, thought and feeling. Phenomenological language and concepts are especially suitable for pursuing the subject of the emotional significance of flesh, and the therapeutic touching of persons, because bodily being is positioned at the outset of discussion. Whatever we perceive, think, feel or do, such activity is firstly and immediately experiential and body-dependant.

Abram (1997) shows that phenomenologists view scientific theory and practice as arising out of directly felt and lived experience. This direct experience continues to sustain science, which therefore has value and meaning only in reference to this primordial, open and experiential realm:

> *'If this body is my very presence in the world, if it is the body that alone enables me to enter into relations with other presences, if without these eyes, this voice or these hands I would be unable to see, to taste, and to touch things, or to be touched by them — if without this body, in other words, there would be no possibility of experience — then the body itself is the true subject of experience.'* (Abram 1997, p 45)

The essential point is that the usual way in which the body is studied and considered is not how it really is. A body as it really is is a body as it experiences and animates itself and its worlds:

> *'...my sadness is indistinguishable from a certain heaviness of my bodily limbs, or as my delight is only artificially separable from the widening of my eyes, from the bounce in my step and the heightened sensitivity of my skin.'* (Abram 1997, p 46)

The body is always a *means*; this is its phenomenological status. It can never be a fully explicit thing because such a description would involve a change in this status. Leder (1992) explains further:

> *'If one notion can be said to lie at the heart of this paradigm, it is that the lived body is an "tending" entity...mean[ing] simply that it is bound up with, and directed toward, an experienced world. It is a being in relationship to that which is other: other people, other things, an environment. Moreover, in a significant sense, the lived body helps to constitute this world-as-experienced. We cannot understand the meaning and form of objects without reference to the bodily powers through which we engage them — our senses, motility, language,*

desires. The lived body is not just one thing in the world, but a way in which the world comes to be...an intentional entity which gives rise to a world.' (Leder 1992, p 25)

The lived body, then, is essentially 'not-only-mechanical'. Instead of regarding the body as a corpse animated by energy or by soul (for example), it should be regarded instead as a body which is the locus of its own world relations. Therefore the physiological is always viewed as 'intertwined with, and an expression of, the body's intentionality' (Leder 1992, p 25). Leder goes on to suggest that a medicine of the lived body dwells in this intertwining, and as such must address the lived body and its world relations (Leder 1992, p 29). According to phenomenology, a given medical condition would need to be described with reference to the sufferer's experienced world. By definition, then, the emotional life of the body-subject at once becomes of great importance in evaluation and the planning of treatment.

Leder gives an example of a hypertensive patient who is:

'...involved in a difficult marriage and job situation. The sense of limitation and frustration which are a daily reality lead, not only to a clenched fist, a sore neck, but to a constricting of the arteries. The patient inhabits, as we might say, a constricted world, and this constriction expresses itself through both surface and visceral musculature. So, too, the temporality of her life-world. Perhaps she is the impatient sort, always rushing to finish projects and make her next appointment. In her struggle to compress time, even her visceral functions — breathing, heartbeat — become compressed and accelerated in ways that can lead to dysfunction.' (Leder 1992, p 28)

It can immediately be seen that this description is of the same kind used by Keleman, Kepner and others offering approaches to body-centred psychology. It may be that this perspective has the advantage of providing a genuinely integrative framework for what has hitherto been only incompletely described as lip service to 'treating the whole person', or addressing 'mind, body and spirit'. Instead of having a variety of concepts such as bio- psycho- social-, somehow in need of effective integration, the body is the ground, the focus of attention, and intentionality is viewed as necessarily embodied, enacted and determined in it.

Clearly, it is not unrealistic to consider blood vessel musculature as capable of responding similarly to somatic musculature. There is no reason why the phenomenon of muscular tension should not occur in blood vessels and other visceral effector systems. But the point is that whilst phenomenology acknowledges traditional Cartesian scientific learning, it refuses to grant it ruling status when describing a patient's condition. Instead, emphasis is placed upon the directly lived patient's world and how this manifests in his 'lived body'. The physiological description is therefore placed in a wider and more usual perspective of living experience. The patient's manner of living, therefore, becomes also his manner of bodily being.

The phenomenological view is much more likely to place importance upon value-laden descriptions of bodily posture ('shouldering the world's burdens' etc) specifically because it argues that they are, in any case, better ways of describing reality. To live as burdened would necessitate the embodiment of burden, its physical expression. An interesting outcome of this use of phenomenological language is that the principle of bodily motility/mobility — or lack of — might emerge as the essential descriptive paradigm in manual therapy. Movement is an idea intimately connected with life and active being-in-the-world. But *tense* shoulder muscles, *constricted* arterial muscle, *taut* intestinal wall muscles — *rigidified* structures in general are all embodiments of a restricted world. The verbs are all negative qualifications of movements; qualifications which express the patient's life intentionality. Restrictions in mobility have occurred — the manual practitioner's frequent concern. A phenomenological investigation into manual therapy diagnosis could consist in an account of how the lived body typically, kinetically expresses and embodies experience in palpable flesh.

The lived body therefore becomes the focus of clinical and philosophical attention. Practitioners of manual therapy are manipulating *incorporated*, sedimented psychological history, enacted interpersonal relations — as well as the site where biological mechanisms are homeostatically maintained (Leder 1992, p 30). Necessarily, practitioners are influencing these non-mechanical worlds, interacting directly with them as world-in-body, as well as with body-in-the-world.

The notion of the lived body holds that there are no purely mechanical disorders, and hence no purely mechanical benefits. Beneficial therapy, according to this theory, would somehow change how the lived body is lived. It would change the intentional world-in-body. The practitioner's project is the relief of a person's discomfort and disability, which, by the phenomenological account are lived and expressed somatically. Since the lived body is a way in which the world comes to be, then the practice of manual therapy might contribute to the alteration of the possibilities for engaging in the world-as-experienced. Freer mobility experienced by the patient doesn't make the patient feel better, rather, it is part of that feeling of betterness.

The change in focus of attention which the concept of the lived-body requires, locates the effects of our experience of life and our intention actually in the body itself, and attributes to the body the ability to express this phenomenological world somatically — especially through musculature. This raises the importance, significance and potency of bodily contact in therapy to hitherto unrecognised heights. As a starting point for a new exploration of manual therapy rationale, the phenomenological paradigm of the lived body seems fertile ground.

The absent body

The phenomenological account of embodiment has produced a further relevant concept. Leder, in *The Absent Body* (1990), shows how certain features of the lived body prevent it from being easily thematised as an experiencing subject. He claims the body is characterised by absence and has intrinsic tendencies towards self-concealment. This follows from the notion that the body is a 'means to other'; whether it is perceptive or motor systems that are being used, they are disclosing the world or acting upon it. So one perceives with and through organs, but one does not perceive the organ perceiving. Similarly, motor activities are performed by various organ clusters, *to* another subject. My attention is not on my legs as I take a free kick, it is wholly upon the ball, whereupon my automatic self organises my body. It is the precise fact that those organs are performing *to* what is other from the body which causes them to disappear. Because the attention is upon the object of endeavours, those engaged bodily activities, as used, are not in focus. Leder enlarges considerably and with sophistication upon this theme, which, in its wider implications, is a significant insight into the study of embodiment.

The significance of the absent body argument is that, in normal life's seamless existence of perception, motility and abstract thought, the body is taken for granted and unnoticed in its natural, unimpaired operation. This means that any notion of the body being lived, as being the seat of distributed mentality, does not easily suggest itself. That is, these features of bodily function both encourage unhelpful dualism and cause the mental significance of flesh to be hidden.

By contrast, when fatigued, perceptually errant, disturbed, inordinately passionate, insane, ill, diseased, or even just emphasised through change, the body is at once placed to the attention of the person as something to be ordinated, calmed, resisted, examined and repaired. In this way it becomes both associated strongly with negativity and also otherness-from-self because it appears in opposition to autonomy, will and understanding (Leder 1990, p 132):

'Insofar as the body seizes our awareness particularly at times of disturbance, it can come to appear "Other" and opposed to the self.'
(Leder 1990, p 70)

For example, in the case of pain, whenever the body perceives itself, an element of distance is introduced. If the perceived event is of high magnitude, its degree of otherness is likewise increased. If the perceived event is unpleasant, distance may seem desirable. This partially accounts for patients' routine descriptions of pain and a painful area as 'it', and as the painful body as 'drawing attention to itself'.

With problematic functioning of either perception, affect, or motility, it can become quite a project to rid oneself of bodily feelings. This is obvious in the case of pain, but less so in emotion such as anxiety, for example, when one becomes aware of heartbeat, choking voice, etc. These events threaten performance and effective functioning in general — even more so if one concentrates on it — so that it becomes necessary to eliminate the feelings. If effective functioning involves not being self-conscious, then attending to the body is likely to disrupt functioning further (Leder 1990, p 85). Whether the feeling is anger, anxiety, pain or any other, the principle is the same; it often seems desirable to eliminate feelings. The point is that if effected, such desire suppresses the body as self-informer, ground of knowledge and therefore as *self*. The negative context of these self-reflections is felt in the body, and the body and its passions become identified with negativity. Thus there is a cultural tendency to render problematic bodily disturbances as negative, or bad, rather than sometimes as informative, educational, and self-revelatory. If this is true, as many suspect it to be, then it can only point to a fundamentally flawed perception of the 'constitution of man'.

The unreasonably great importance attached to freedom-from-problematic functioning encourages unreasonable attempts at self-detachment, distancing and non-identification with the dysfunctioning body. This is in addition to those attempts to quash such feelings without first placing them in their deserved existential context. This may be especially true of emotional discomfort. The compelling nature of emotions (one cannot close them down as one can close one's eyes) renders the soul or mind as passive — out of control, even, in the face of a lust threatening to disrupt moral behaviour. This too has a distancing effect from the self and may lead to emotional suppression. This time it is not merely because the emotions may be unpleasant (especially in a social context), but because they appear to have a *life of their own*, that is, they may feel non-self. Viscera can reflect emotions — especially strong ones. A chronically tense person, for example, may show increased stomach acid secretion, but the gut will not respond to command as will certain groupings of muscles. This inability to control the viscera will encourage poor correlation of self with viscera (Leder 1990, p 50), which are mediators of emotion. The divorcement of the self from the passions, in favour of the higher mind or intellect, further discourages inclusion of the body under the category of self. An absent body, after all, might be a more effective one.

If this description of bodily absence is convincing, then it explains why notions such as body-memory, psychogenic bodily morbid change, in fact any aspect of the body as lived, have failed to present themselves as conspicuous themes in human biology. Moreover, the apparent objectivity and otherness of the body has served to emphasise machine-like automaticity and has equated emotion with it. Has all this been encouraged by a negative attitude towards dysfunction, illness and passion, and an obsession with control and efficiency?

Value has tended to be placed upon a disembodied state, equating it with the soul and its self. The body and *its* self have remained a largely denied force, concealed by the social attitude towards its own beautiful efficiency.

Phenomenology probably represents the cutting edge of conceptual philosophy in the realm of health care, and is suggesting itself as an accurate and efficacious conceptual framework in the field. It is a practical approach to dispensing with dualism, and to humanising biological and medical science. Manual medicine would do well to explore it, and experiment optimistically with its language forms and its shifts in perspective. As a first suggestion, the use of the word 'touch' would, if it were allowed to infiltrate the explanations and narratives used in manual therapy, invoke the experiential and emotional domains — the 'phenomenal' world — so absent from its current literature.

Phenomenology — conclusions

Touching is never merely a mechanical act because the agent and recipient are, as it were, attitudinally loaded with respect to interpersonal transactions of any sort. The more one tries to pretend that human beings are machines, the more practitioners' and patients' psychological lives are ignored, suppressed and excluded from healing processes. Yet the appropriate nurturing of these may be the most efficacious facilitator of healing.

Touching is never merely a mechanical act because flesh is not inanimate material. Flesh is that which gives rise to activity and allows perception. Flesh is both objective and subjective. It is the 'I' as it makes contact with the world. Any attempt to analyse flesh without its 'I' will result in an atypical description — a description which is artificial, uncommon and unreal. Flesh as seen without its 'I' is not how flesh is. Flesh is lived.

However, the baby must not be lost just because some bath water is being drained away. The mechanistic tool of manual therapy has much validation on a mechanical and physiological level. This is not to be denied, but merely placed in a more realistic context. Flesh may well be 'lived', but it is also *of the earth* and therefore willingly succumbs to a certain degree of material analysis.

THE OMISSION OF THE STUDY OF TOUCH

Although it is obvious that practitioners of manual medicine, manipulation, massage and other bodywork touch and handle their patients, nevertheless the subject of touch is omitted from the majority of curricula. It is true that touch is covered in massage teachings to some degree, but it is notable in orthodox manipulation — chiropractic, osteopathy and physiotherapy — by its absence. It is not difficult to see why this is the case. For example, a fairly recent well-respected text in osteopathic diagnosis, in a chapter entitled 'The Philosophy of Osteopathic Medicine' (Martinke 1989) includes the following summary of osteopathic principles:

1. The body is a unit.
2. Structure and function are reciprocally inter-related.
3. The body possesses self-regulatory mechanisms.
4. The body has the inherent capacity to defend and repair itself.
5. When normal adaptability is disrupted, or when environmental changes overcome the body's capacity for self-maintenance, disease may ensue.
6. Movement of body fluids is essential to the maintenance of health.
7. The nerves play a crucial role in controlling the fluids of the body.
8. There are somatic components to disease that are not only manifestations of disease, but are also factors that contribute to maintenance of the diseased state.

It is interesting that none of the above precepts implies what should be done to the patient — none implies that the touching of patients is a therapeutic modality naturally or obviously arising out of it. This suggests that further arguments are necessary to show why osteopaths use touch rather than any other therapeutic modality as the treatment of choice.[1]

Understandably, osteopaths and other manipulators have described their science and art by using concepts of human constitution, body functioning or processes of health and illness. This is quite proper, for without a coherent theory of human constitution, theories of health and illness remain incomplete or confused. Once a reasonable working theory of human constitution is articulated and accepted, health and illness concepts can, in theory, be deduced from it.

But for concepts of healing whereby one (or more) human being heals or attempts to promote healing in another, the subsequent immediate requirement is a coherent theory of practitioner–patient relationship. Since the therapeutic relationship is the setting for the healing arts, it is the ground out of which theories and practices of interactive healing processes will grow. Some examples of partitive (ie emphasising special aspects of) theories of relationship are those explored by Balint (1974), Neighbour (1987), Reilly (1996), Latey (1997a, b), and of course the mass of literature concerning psychotherapeutic models.

So the prerequisite concepts underlying all therapeutics (save self-healing) are human *constitution* and *relationships*.

Constitution

As is well-known, orthodox medicine, which includes manipulative medicine, identifies human constitution as very largely mechanical in nature. This book seeks to add, in its own way, a psychological component to this identity. A great many other texts of studies in holistic medical subjects have done the same. That a psychological–physical human should be placed in his or her familial and social context for the purposes of evaluation and assistance is also familiar to good practitioners.

But a theory of constitution will need to include energetics, field theory, subtle-body theory, spirituality and even theosophy if it is to satisfy the current inclinations in the development of our understanding of the human condition. Theories of these kinds are as immature and varied as theories of biological functioning were 200 years ago. The reason they should be researched and taken seriously is that they provide the only possibility for a comprehensive understanding of human life — one that explicitly allows for the wealth of history of human experience.

There are a great many models of psychological constitution, some of which are mentioned in this book. They will be useful in providing a wider context in which to place the more limited mechanical and physiological theories of constitution. But the sheer number and variation of psychological models poses a problem to those who would synthesise a comprehensive constitutional model. Naturally enough, the response to this is often that different models suit different people at different times, for different purposes. This is very true, but there should at least be some possibility of integrating conflicting proposals. Psychological constitutional theory alone would have to account for:

- emotional phenomena, which appear very much to be associated with soma
- intellectual phenomena, which may appear less associated with soma but which are no less capable of influencing healing
- volitional phenomena, which are also distinct
- spiritual phenomena, which although controversial, have nevertheless dominated human life since records of it began.

The challenges created and the questions posed by reducing the role of physiology in manual therapy are numerous and complicated. This book leads to the inescapable fact that Pandora's box of somatic psychology is wide open. And the puzzle of emotion and flesh begs the question of the wider issues involved in understanding human constitution. A further problem may be that psychological models themselves tend to be studied in a way which purports to be scientific. This very attempt to objectify subjectivity may actually fail to notice its beauty and depth.

Thus it can be seen that human constitutional theory is, in reality, in a neonatal state. Universally accepted concepts exist only in the realms of physiology, and to a considerably smaller extent in the realms of emotionology (despite what psychologists lead one to believe) and other less corporeal disciplines.

Relationship

Bearing the foregoing in mind, thus far there exist some very useful theories of how manual therapy may promote healing in irritated, fatigued or damaged human tissue. That is, the nature of the therapeutic relationship on a mechanical level is reasonably well understood. But relationships are usually understood in psychological terms. So because the influence of psychological processes upon physiological ones in general and healing in particular is so great, then psychological processes in relationships are profoundly important to all medicine, including manual therapy. Again, the difficulty may then lie in the choice of psychological models available, and the suspicion that the existence of a large number of these suggests a fair degree of inaccuracy in each. Accuracy in conflicting physiological theories is reconciled by scientific research of the sort which is unavailable to psychology. Psychology as it is currently understood simply does not lend itself to traditional scientific study. Variety in psychology will therefore persist unless a universally accepted philosophical context emerges for its analysis. A new tolerance of philosophical method is necessary for this to proceed.

The importance of touch lies in its being at the synapse — literally the interface of a manual therapy relationship. It is where the practitioner meets the patient on the plane of bodily proximity — intimacy. Indeed, touch appears to be the essence or epitome of the therapeutic relationship. It is what manual practitioners *do*. But it is vital to notice that touch is also the embodiment of certain important aspects of the emotional relationship between practitioner and patient. The evidence for this has been presented in this book.

In the field of manual therapy, therefore, a consideration of the subject of touch follows naturally from a consideration of relationship. Under the generic heading of therapeutic relationship, touch is the species which contains the potential for the most powerful blend of physical and emotional healing processes. Because manual practitioners have not studied what they do from the point of view of interpersonal relationship, the concept of touch has never arisen. It has simply never emerged as a subject worthy of study in its own right. This is precisely because touch is something that people do to each other, whereas manipulation is seen as something people do to bodies. In other words this situation has arisen out of inaccurate models of constitution and therapeutic relationship. Healing concepts must begin with relationship, in the knowledge of constitution. Only then can they look at therapeutic modality.

Constitution plus *relationship* informs *therapy*. This being the case, shattering the belief that manual therapy is only a mechanophysiological discipline opens the door to extraordinarily creative possibilities.

ETHICAL ISSUES AND THE WAY FORWARD

It should be reaffirmed that ethics are involved in each and every clinical interaction because it is not possible to distinguish ethical problems from non-ethical problems in medical care interactions (Seedhouse 1991). Ethical issues concern all interpersonal behaviour. Therefore ethical issues in manual therapy may differ only in certain respects from those in non-manual interactions, for example as a result of the degree of intimacy involved in the former. In other words, because ethics involve how one ought to behave in the presence of others, and since touching involves behaving directly *onto* others, then certain ethical considerations are inevitably larger (the fact that, in the UK, the law considers intentional touching without permission to be assault, reflects this). Ethical issues in psychologically significant manual therapy are perhaps a step yet more intense.

In this brief exposure of the intimacy of the therapeutic encounter, at this early stage in the evolution of manual therapy, there are special issues in ethics which need to be brought out. These can be summarised by saying that in proportion as a practitioner enters into more authentic, current and complex relationships with patients, then accordingly he has many more issues of an ethical nature to consider. These will be partly those ethical issues debated within the psychotherapy and counselling professions, and they will, naturally, centre around the relationship between patients and their practitioners.

This book has merely exposed the misrepresentation which has befallen manual therapy. It is not intended as a guide for practice and others must step in to provide this. The ethical issues which will emerge as the professions develop their understanding and change their behaviour will need to be aired with honesty, humility and care. Some general points arise at the conclusion of this text.

Transference

One of the most interesting subjects concerns the use of transference, and this was mentioned at the end of the previous chapter. Broadly speaking there are two opposing views:

[handwritten margin note: Both are true ideas / there are for both]

1. Parent/adult type relationships between patients and practitioners are actually necessary in order to cause resolution of certain body-self disorders and this should be recognised and utilised.

2. Parent/adult type relationships, in addition to other 'nuclear family' type relationships, are inherently unhealthy and need to be avoided for health to prevail.

The first view makes explicit use of the need by some patients to be cared for when they feel unable to cope adequately themselves. It also implies acceptance of the use of power in relationship, and the recognition that patients may at times be relating to practitioners from child-like mental positions or 'ego-states'. The second emphasises patient autonomy and independence and strives to facilitate their emergence from the start; the patient is encouraged to use an adult ego-state when interacting with the practitioner. In the exploration of the problem of transference, the special issues of the use of power in paternalistic models of healing, and the place of autonomy within such schemes, need to be aired.

It must be emphasised here that the view by the majority is that transference occurs in every case where there is a patient/practitioner interaction, and especially so where the patient disrobes and is handled by the practitioner. It is almost inevitable that patients will not see practitioners as ordinary human beings, but as special ones. At times this may be useful — necessary, even. At others it will be unhelpful, possibly even damaging. What is vital is that practitioners realise this, understand it, and learn how best to deal with any difficulties that may arise as a result of it.

Patient education

It is one thing to recognise and try to understand the psychodynamics of relationship and its potential for healing. It is another to recognise that flesh is emotionally alive and that its form represents sedimented psychoemotional history. Both these concepts are relevant to any healing relationship. But the latter informs especially those therapeutics which address the patient with physical directness. This is because it exposes manual bodywork as *person-work*, and because it allows for a richer exploration of the psychological and emotional causes of ill-health.

If, for example, the Frankl–Randell theory of psychosomatic biopathy is correct and practitioners are educated to understand the hypnotic basis of their manipulations, should they still offer (false) mechanical explanations to their patients? Should the reality of the lived body be educated to patients? If so it is hoped that the consequences would be improved and more complete self-knowledge, self-awareness and autonomy, resulting in a vastly improved capacity for self-care. But in the absence of a sensitive and thoughtful empathic practitioner as agent, the consequences might be pain, guilt and confusion. This might arise as a result of the degree to which inaccurate theories of constitution, health and illness pervade the fabric of Western thought processes. That is, the making explicit of what has been so strongly denied at such a fundamental somatopsychic level is a complex and difficult task. Overall, it must be right to educate and inform because the creation of autonomy is perhaps the most useful over-riding ethical principle (Seedhouse 1988).

Interprofessional collaboration

The insights of manual practitioners have much to offer bodyworking and other psychotherapists. This is because in palpating the form and quality of static and moving tissue to such an exquisitely fine degree, manual practitioners are feeling the patient's very emotional autobiography, the patient's self as embodied. Manual practitioners can provide important insights into patterns of embodiment, systems of tension, types of constricted tissue. They should be able to map the changes in tissue that have taken place in an individual and use this as a potent source of information to be used in healing environments and relationships.

The insights of psychology have much to offer manual therapists. They provide an understanding of the hitherto denied aspect of their patients, an aspect which is essential to each patient's body-self. They provide a better partitive understanding of the person than an exploration of flesh does. They offer the human form an emotional architecture, a lived significance.

Defining boundaries of expertise

Encouraging the cognitive participation of patients in their healing, where problems have been of an emotional nature, may cross boundaries with psychotherapy. This is a very difficult area, and will have to be a matter for intercourse and definition within the professions. For who is to say that communication which is mature, compassionate, sensitive and reasonable is not valuable and right in any relationship? If a practitioner untrained in standard psychotherapeutic techniques or counselling nevertheless engages in this kind of communication with her patient, how does she define her level of expertise? Who is to say what is and what is not such and such a therapy, when the relationship between practitioner and patient is more important than its apparent context. This is the crunch: tools (therapies) are likely to be significantly less important than relationship. But the tool is the vehicle upon which the relationship begins its ride. The tool of touch, more than any other, immediately and dramatically places the relationship in a emotionally and existentially significant context.

What practitioners do with this knowledge (of relationship, and of flesh as the emotionally alive body-self) is in need of very careful study indeed. To remain tied only to physiological and neurological reflex-type theories may be delusion, if one continues to practise in the same way as before. Either one should stick to physiological theories only and treat tissue damage, or one should accept that manual therapy is unconsciously psychologically significant, and that psychological processes are playing an important — possibly vital and major — part in what is assumed to be a mechanical/physiological process.

The way forward is to widen the therapeutic rationale of manual therapy to include a psychological view of fleshly matters, so that it is explicit that bodywork is to do with healing whole selves. In doing this, there are two extreme positions on a continuum of possibilities. Practitioners could remain merely *aware* of the importance of emotion in manual therapy, and change their practical approach only in accordance with the effect of such awareness. Or else the special understanding of the human condition revealed by knowledge of body-self and its processes should be used to advance the actual form which manual therapy takes in practice.

Both options would progress the science and art of manual therapy in a way which is realistic, more accurate and whole, in proportion as it researches and integrates psychosomatic understanding. Both these developments would create increased maturity in the patient–practitioner relationship. Furthermore, both would, in theory, decrease the potential for the abuse of patients. This is because contained in the subtle and compassionate psychological understanding of patients is also an understanding of how they become needy, vulnerable and unhealthily dependent upon carers, and how these situations might be avoided. Similarly, these developments would protect against the tendency of carers to become unsatisfied, overworked or bored. This would arise out of a richer understanding of the dynamics of patient–practitioner relationship, and how these might become optimally efficient and fulfilling for both parties. Practitioners would, quite simply, have to examine their procedures and transactions in considerably more detail than they may currently feel obliged to do. After all, working with a real person is rather more ethically loaded than mending a broken object.

In either case, in being educated in matters of the psychological meaning of bodily form and quality, practitioners must be as equally educated in psychology and transference matters to the degree that they are capable of avoiding: unwittingly abusing patients; causing uncontainable catharsis; creating overdependence; and generally bringing out patients' emotional issues and then not being able to help to contain them. Naturally, self-reflection, introspection and examination of practitioners' own characters and needs would be necessary. This would be partly to examine how practitioners' own feelings towards their patients influence their work. The more practitioners feel the need to change their mode of practice, the more heightened the need for ethical awareness, supervision, research, and professional debate.

The advancement in manual therapy that would occur if its therapeutic rationale were to be widened as suggested might pose what could be called 'a challenge of excellence' for the profession. At the outset, a more explicit consideration of the emotional dimension of somatic biopathy, if not undertaken extremely carefully, might cause a rise in ethical difficulties encountered by the profession. This would occur if practitioners' abilities to contain the more human problems (as opposed to merely mechanical ones) which would emerge in practice did not match that very emergence. However, because the widened rationale would specifically promote a more humanistic perspective, then practitioners would in fact be better placed to:

- understand and contain the problems posed by emotionally vulnerable patients, through the consideration of them from within a more satisfactory theoretical base, and the gaining of insight into the special patterns of relating that they exhibit
- take precautions to ensure that misunderstandings, undue dependencies and other difficulties do not occur, and be able to make better problem-solving decisions when they do
- reflect more effectively upon their work and satisfaction with professional life.

In the presence of a suitable postgraduate, professional development structure involving supervision, these effects would be enhanced. Such an institution would foster:

- improvement in the long-term effectiveness of practitioners
- regular reflection upon practitioners' general and emotional health, work contentment and personal needs in the working context
- regular reflection upon professional needs
- more ethical work.

Unquestionably, one of the results of such endeavour would be an improvement in the quality of patients' feelings and beliefs that they are being effectively, properly and well cared for. As stated above, this would be reflected in a corresponding decrease in patient dissatisfaction and a decrease in complaints made against practitioners. It would, in addition, be reflected in a greater need for services.

There is, clearly, a need for a great deal more work. This means work in the realms of clinical relationships — especially those where touching is used — in the reconciliation of the various psychological and constitutional models, and in the realms of psychosomatic and somatopsychic processes. Those practitioners who feel that, for their purposes, the purely physiological rationale underlying manual therapy is a sufficient one, will need to confine themselves explicitly to the treatment of self-evidently mechanical tissue damage. There

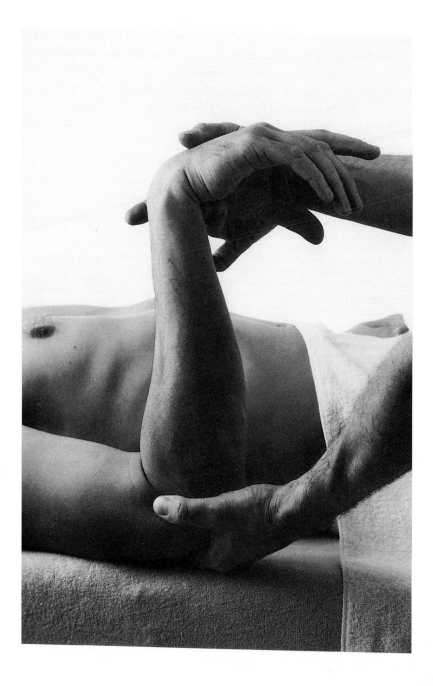

is nothing whatever wrong in this, so long as practitioners are aware of the limitations in explanation and expertise imposed by this view. But to continue to practise manipulative or manual therapy under the impression that its wonderful effects are of a purely mechanical nature is simply to deny the reality of the situation, and actively to stagnate the science and art of healing.

NOTES

[1]It should be noted that this particular text reflects the attitude towards osteopathic philosophy in North America, where osteopathy has been absorbed into mainstream medicine, and thus surgical and pharmacological intervention are considered within a framework of osteopathic philosophy. Such intervention is thus deemed 'osteopathic', and so these authors need not take pains to point toward manipulation as the natural therapeutic modality. The attitude and medical political situation in Great Britain is quite different, and although manipulation is the *sine qua non* of British osteopathy (and is largely carried out by practitioners not trained in the mainstream medical system), to my knowledge no osteopathic philosophical precepts have been articulated which self-evidently and naturally conclude with the need for manual therapy.

REFERENCES

Abram D 1997 The spell of the sensuous: perception and meaning in a more than human world. Vintage, New York

Balint M 1974 The doctor, his patient and the illness. Pitman, London

Latey P J 1997a Basic clinical tactics. Journal of Bodywork and Movement Therapies 1(3): 163–172

Latey P J 1997b The balance of practice: preparing for long-term work. Journal of Bodywork and Movement Therapies 1(4): 223–230

Leder D 1990 The absent body. University of Chicago Press, Chicago

Leder D 1992 A tale of two bodies: the Cartesian corpse and the lived body. In: Leder D (ed) The body in medical thought and practice. Philosophy and Medicine Series, vol 43, Kluwer Academic Publishers, Dordrecht, p 17–36

Martinke D J 1989 The philosophy of osteopathic medicine. In: An osteopathic approach to diagnosis and treatment. Lippincott, New York

Neighbour R 1987 The inner consultation. MTP Press (Kluwer Academic Publishers), Dordrecht

Reilly D 1996 Creating therapeutic consultations. Audiotape of lecture given at conference. The Placebo Response: Biology and Belief, University of Westminster, London (Tapes available from the Scientific and Medical Network, UK)

Seedhouse D 1988 Ethics: the heart of health care. Wiley, Chichester

Seedhouse D 1991 Editorial: Against medical ethics: a philosopher's view. Medical Education 25: 280–282

Index